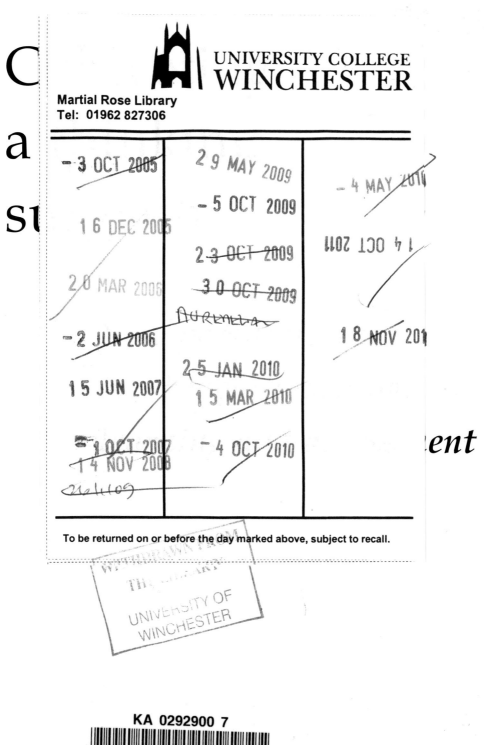

Cultivating a thinking surgeon

New perspectives on clinical teaching, learning and assessment

Linda de Cossart ChM FRCS
Consultant Vascular Surgeon
Countess of Chester NHS Foundation Trust

Della Fish MA MEd PhD Dip Ed
Professor of Education (postgraduate medicine)
King's College, London
Education Adviser to Kent, Surrey and Sussex Deanery
for postgraduate medical and dental education

tfm Publishing Ltd, Castle Hill Barns, Harley, Nr Shrewsbury, SY5 6LX, UK.
Tel: +44 (0)1952 510061; Fax: +44 (0)1952 510192
E-mail: nikki@tfmpublishing.com; Web site: www.tfmpublishing.com

Design and layout: Nikki Bramhill

Printed by Gutenberg Press Ltd., Gudja Road, Tarxien, PLA 19, Malta.

Tel: +356 21897037; Fax: +356 21800069.

If you have responsibilities for teaching you must develop the skills, attitudes and practices of a competent teacher. You must also make sure that students and junior colleagues are properly supervised.

General Medical Council (GMC), (2001) *Good Medical Practice.* London: GMC
(No: 16 of the duties of a doctor)

The conditions necessary for a surgeon are four: first, he should be learned. Second, he should be expert. Third, he must be ingenious. Fourth, he should be able to adapt himself.

Guy de Chauliac. *The Art of Surgery* 1363
The first European book on surgery

Shah, Z. (2003) 'Endpiece', *British Medical Journal*, 327, 29th Nov 2003,
p. 1263.

Contents

Résumé and implications

Figures and tables

Glossary

A&E	Accident and Emergency
BERA	British Educational Research Association
BST	Basic Surgical Training
CA	Conversation Analysis
CCT	Certificate of Completion of Training
CCST	Certificate of Completion of Specialist Training
CT scan	Computerized Tomography scan
CV	Curriculum Vitae
EU	European Union
EWTD	European Working Time Directive
F1	Foundation Year One
F2	Foundation Year Two
FRCS	Fellow of the Royal College of Surgeons
GMC	General Medical Council
GP	General Practitioner
GPPS	The General Professional Practice of Surgery (the draft curriculum for surgical SHOs)
HIV	Human Immuno-deficiency Virus
MD	Doctor of Medicine
MESB	Medical Education Standards Board
MMC	Modernising Medical Careers
MS	Master of Surgery
MRSA	Methicillin-resistant *Staphylococcus aureus*
NHS	National Health Service
ODP	Operating Department Practitioner
OED	Oxford English Dictionary

PA	Professional Artistry (mindset of a professional)
PGMDE	Post Graduate Medical and Dental Education
PhD	Doctor of Philosophy
PMETB	Postgraduate Medical Education and Training Board
RCS Eng	The Royal College of Surgeons of England
RITA	Record of In-service Training Assessment
SET	Schedule for Evaluating Teaching
SHO	Senior House Officer
SpR	Specialist Registrar
STEPS	Schedule for the Evaluation of Problem Solving
STOPS	Schedule for the Evaluation of Psycho-motor Skills
TA	Triggered Assessment
TR	Technical Rational (mindset of a professional)
UK	United Kingdom

Acknowledgements

Formal thanks are due to the Royal College of Surgeons of England for permission to use extracts from several college documents relating to the *draft* curriculum for surgical SHOs; and to the Ursula Keys Fund, which has funded the Chester Multi-disciplinary Theatre Team Project.

We are also grateful to: Professor Colin Coles for helpful suggestions in refining the elements of clinical thinking as well as considerable encouragement and support; Brenda Owen-Jones, Practice Development Nurse at The Countess of Chester NHS Foundation Trust for permission to use the first page of her in-house log-book for First Assistants in Theatre; Professor Michael Golby for oral and written ideas as acknowledged in the text, as well as for continued inspiration about many matters educational; Suzanne Gorne (surgical SHO) for making the point that clinical solutions come in the plural rather than the singular; and members of many of our seminars and workshops who have seized upon our developing thinking and helped us to refine it further.

We particularly thank the following, without whom we could not have begun let alone completed this enterprise, and who have helped us in many ways:

- ❒ Our colleagues in Trusts (particularly The Countess of Chester NHS Foundation Trust, and other Trusts in Merseyside and the South of England) whose practice has inspired our thinking and who are wise enough to recognize that there is more to being a good doctor than just toiling away at clinical processes and procedures. We thank them for providing us with evidence to support our ideas; for being brave enough to explore them for themselves in practice; for challenging how we express them; for turning our thinking into reality; and for being concerned enough to give us honest and sensible critiques.
- ❒ Our educational colleagues and all the committed surgeon and physician educators in Kent, Surrey and Sussex Deanery, and the deaneries of Mersey and Wessex, who have sustained and encouraged us in the struggle to clarify and articulate what is involved in the practice of education, and who share with us a concern about the quality of what is currently being offered to postgraduate doctors in the name of training.
- ❒ Our respective friends and family who have missed time with us because of our new venture, but who we hope will be proud of it.
- ❒ Key consultants and teachers in our lives in whom we have seen the meaning of true professional practice in the way they have attended to both the humanitarian and specialist aspects of their work.

❏　Bright-eyed and idealistic learners who will be the leaders of surgery of the future and who will be let down by the system if we do not provide ways of developing how they can best be taught, and whose interests we wished to serve by having them in our sights while writing.

❏　Members of the Chester Multi-disciplinary Theatre Team Project, who have given us further evidence that the commitment to good teaching as well as good surgical standards of practice is alive and well. The project has confirmed our belief that even the most difficult challenges are fun, rewarding and professionally motivating, and that there is a huge resource in clinical practice waiting to be led towards richer approaches to education.

❏　Jean Douglas and Evelyn Usher, our intrepid proof readers, who have saved us from numerous errors and helped us to achieve the most elegant prose of which we are capable, and in defence of whom we must say that any remaining mistakes of any kind are assuredly ours and not theirs.

❏　Nikki Bramhill and tfm publishing Ltd., for taking on the task of offering our ideas to the world at large, and for making the process smooth and enjoyable.

Please note: the ideas contained in this publication are our own and are not necessarily shared by any institutions for which we work.

About the authors

Linda de Cossart

Linda graduated in medicine from the University of Liverpool in 1972, determined to follow a career in surgery. Her postgraduate career started in Liverpool and led to teaching anatomy at Liverpool and at the University of Texas. She obtained a Masters in Surgery on the subject of Tissue Plasminogen Activator in Venous Disease at Liverpool in 1983. Her clinical career followed the traditional pattern of the day and as a Registrar at Hope Hospital, Manchester and Aintree Hospital, Liverpool she gained a wide experience in clinical surgery. As a Senior Registrar in Chester and Broadgreen Hospital, Liverpool she consolidated her clinical expertise before becoming a Consultant in Vascular and General Surgery at Chester in 1988. One of her roles at that time was as President of the Association of Surgeons in Training.

Her consultant career as a General and Vascular Surgeon began with a wide remit including urological surgery and involved developing research in venous disease as well as pioneering networked vascular emergency cover. As Associate Postgraduate Dean and Programme Director in General Surgery, she has been able to influence both the organizational and the educational aspects of surgical education and training. She has been a member of the Specialist Advisory Committee in General Surgery, Secretary of the Vascular Surgical Society, and was elected to the Council of The Royal College of Surgeons of England in 1999. Her interest in surgical education has existed throughout her career and is now underpinned by not only theoretical concepts but a wide clinical experience. She was invited to give the Royal College of Surgeons of England's Moynihan Lecture in 2005.

Della Fish

Della graduated in English in 1965, completed a postgraduate teaching certificate in 1966 and joined the staff of Marlborough Grammar School. She subsequently gained an MA, and then a PhD, both in English Renaissance poetry, and later an MEd in Curriculum Design and Development.

Between 1969 and 1994 she worked in Teacher Education, with both undergraduates and postgraduates, returning to the school classroom at various stages during this period. She joined the Education Department of West London Institute of Higher Education (later incorporated into Brunel University) in 1980, where she became Principal Lecturer. Alongside her main roles in teacher education, she supported occupational therapy staff in designing a new diploma and degree programme, and was rapidly drawn into working with educators in occupational therapy, physiotherapy and nursing. A developing passion for the challenge of providing education in clinical settings led her, in 1994, to extend this work into a full time consultancy which supports educators in almost every health care profession. In 1999 she began work in medical education, as an educational adviser to South Thames Deanery, and now works for Kent, Surrey and Sussex Deanery. Between 2000 and 2003, Della worked for the Royal College of Surgeons of England, with Linda, in developing the draft curriculum for SHOs in surgery. In late 2003 she joined the Institute of Learning and Teaching at King's College, London with a Chair in Education (postgraduate medicine), and currently co-directs with Linda, the Chester Multi-disciplinary Theatre Project. She is the external examiner for a masters degree in Advanced Clinical Practice at the University of Wales, Swansea.

Della's last three books (Fish and Twinn, 1997; Fish and Coles, 1998; and Fish, 1998), have focused on teaching and learning in clinical settings. She has contributed two chapters on practice knowledge in health care to Higgs *et al*, (2004); and her chapter on educational evaluation for clinical supervisors will appear in Rose and Best, (2005). She is currently working on a book on a practice curriculum for medical education with Colin Coles, for the Open University. She also writes poetry.

Introduction

Our intentions for this book

This book is for both teachers and learners in surgical practice. Much of it would also be of interest to all who work in Post Graduate Medical and Dental Education (PGMDE). It is about the *practice* of education as it relates to doctors who work, learn and teach in clinical settings. That is, it is focused on the practice of teaching, learning and assessment, the principles and values that underlie that practice, and their development and refinement. In this sense, it seeks to suggest the sort of standards implicit in the term 'sound educational practice', and to provoke readers either to give grounds for refuting their importance, or to work actively to support and develop them.

It should be remembered, however, that learning 'the practice of education' is itself a lifelong enterprise, and that there is neither a quick fix approach to it, nor a set of recipes that will begin to do it justice. Like all 'practices', it is learnt gradually, by engaging in it mindfully. Learning the practice of education neither springs fully-fledged in the hearts and minds of teachers, nor do they have to have developed all these capabilities perfectly *before* working with learners. The teaching process is professional development for both learner and teacher. A practice is learnt by engaging in it thoughtfully and critically and is illuminated by the ideas of others who are part of the same tradition.

For those who aspire to prepare surgeons of the future in a serious and rigorous way, and those who seek to learn to be well-cultivated, thinking surgeons, we offer this book as a companion along what will be a physically and intellectually challenging and rewarding journey. Our ultimate motivation here is our conviction that improving education is the very best way of improving patient care.

We seek in this publication, then, to provide challenging new perspectives that seriously question much that the current climate of PGMDE promotes. We believe that the time is ripe for crystallizing better ways forward in surgical and medical education. We perceive that currently there is no informed debate about the best ways in which to develop doctors and surgeons during their postgraduate years. Indeed, it seems to us that the voice of education has been submerged in a rush to create speedy solutions to problems that have not been fully analyzed. In contributing some ideas about the practice of education, and seating these in examples of good teaching and learning for surgeons, then, we are attempting to illustrate other ways forward. Our aim is to encourage wise deliberation and consequently sound and logical decisions about matters which will have far reaching effects on health care in the 21st Century.

This book, then, offers the voice of education rather than training. It provides an example of the detailed arguments, ideas, processes and language in which to think and talk about education logically and rationally in order to determine the best basis for carrying it out. We are saddened by the current trend to train rather than educate postgraduate doctors - the more so because this approach is being pressed upon medicine and medical education to the point where it is virtually a *fait accompli*, without considering other approaches, and without any evidence that it is the best way forward. Indeed, it seems to us to arise from misguided notions that trade long-term benefits for short-term quick fixes, and that are unaware of, or ignore, potentially better and more economic approaches.

As authors, we draw upon considerable combined experience in surgery, surgical teaching and educational *practice*. We do not offer undigested educational theory. Rather, we seek to develop in readers an understanding and ultimately a refinement of the educational *practices* in which they engage. We also hope to establish a recognition that for the long-term success of surgical education and ultimately of surgical practice, these educational activities need to be underpinned and unified by sound educational principles and a knowledge of how to choose and defend the kind of education that best suits the successful development of surgeons and the practice of surgery.

We take as our foundation the arguments, values and principles that clarify the nature of education and of educational practice. We have been concerned to shape our educational intentions around the notion of enabling doctors to *become* surgeons and *conduct* themselves as professionals (rather than training them in surgical behaviour). We seek to illuminate the importance of a partnership in learning between the surgeon educator and the learning surgeon, and we treat this and its implications seriously. We take a holistic view of surgical practice, rather than seeing it as something to be atomized into fragments and taught and assessed in bits. That is, we believe that the professional's knowing and doing are all part of one holistic process of thoughtful or intelligent practice (see Ryle, 1949). Here, we subscribe to Gardner's 'Multiple Intelligences' (see Gardner, 1993), and the notion that physicians or surgeons bring to their practice the whole of themselves as human beings, not merely parts of their minds or bodies. Intelligent practice itself, we suggest, is the coming together of 'being, thinking, knowing, doing and extending practice'. And these are underpinned by values, beliefs, assumptions, feelings, and personal theories which for all of us, whether we acknowledge it or not, arise from our entire autobiography and have been shaped by experiences, some of which we may barely remember.

In relation to the evolution of this book, we have adopted the role of practitioner researchers and taken a broadly 'action research' and cyclical approach, which we believe will be evident to the discerning reader. We began by seeking first to explore *in the practice setting* the real everyday complex work of our surgical colleagues (their thinking, knowing and doing). We brought up to that our educational philosophy, modifying our practical ideas and suggestions in the light of their starting points, and adapting these further in response to their reactions to them in the practice setting (how useful they have found them and in what ways). In that sense we model what we are advocating indirectly throughout Part two of this book and directly in its final chapter, namely a practitioner researcher approach to practice (both surgical and educational).

Being a surgeon, then, involves being a professional with all that that means in terms of relating to patients and colleagues and knowing oneself. Engaging in doing which itself is intelligent (thoughtful and knowledgeable) means being aware of the knowledge and clinical thinking that are the bases of one's practice. Developing means engaging in professional development both educationally and surgically. We have attempted to attend to all these and to how they come together in the activity we have characterized as cultivating a surgeon.

We offer these ideas in two parts (as indicated in the contents page), the first of which seeks to establish the *educational foundations* for cultivating a surgeon, the second of which looks in considerable detail at the *practice of education* (including assessment) in surgical settings. All chapters start with a summary of their main contents, in order to help readers to locate ideas and processes that they may wish to consider or re-read.

Through the two parts of the book there are six main themes, which we hope emerge clearly, as follows.

Theme 1: Being/Becoming

This is about the surgeon being and becoming a growing professional.

For example, the new doctor becoming a surgeon or the registrar becoming a consultant is essentially about 'coming to be' rather than simply 'learning to do'. This involves learning to be a member of a profession, being clear about one's own personal and professional values, and gradually taking on a wider view of, and role in, the Trust as an entity and the surgical profession as a whole. We believe that the foundations of all these matters need to be set in motion from the beginning of surgical education (see Chapters 1 and 2).

Theme 2: The practice of education (learning, teaching and assessment)

This is about the thinking, knowing and doing that the teacher and learner need to understand, be committed to and be able to enact, if the enterprise is to count as education.

For example, this includes understanding what makes teaching an educational practice (and in what ways it might fail to be truly educational); what sort of educational values and principles underpin that practice; how to provide a nurturing environment for learners; how to free learners to think for themselves; how to make explicit the tacit knowledge and experience that learners need to access; how to assess that learning so that it educates the learner; and how to engage in reflecting on experience so that the invisible elements of practice are made visible (see Chapters 3 to 6).

Theme 3: Clinical thinking

This is about all the cognitive processes of reasoning, decision-making, deliberating and exercising professional judgement that lie behind the practitioner's 'doing'.

For example, this focuses upon all those cognitive processes which result in a medical action, a clinical decision, or a professional judgement, and the assessment of surgeons' abilities in these (see Chapters 7 and 8).

Theme 4: Knowing

This is about all the different kinds of knowing that surgeons call upon in the course of 'doing', together with their associated and varied ways of seeing the world and of understanding it.

For example, this includes: factual medical knowledge; knowledge about how to do things (formal procedural knowledge and know-how); sensory knowledge; intuitive knowledge; knowledge gained through theorizing practice; knowledge gained through improvisation; tacit knowledge; personal knowledge; and self-knowledge (see Chapter 9).

Theme 5: Doing

This is about nurturing learning surgeons and assessing their success in the operative and technical procedures and the clinical processes that are carried out as activities by the surgeon in the entire clinical setting.

For example, this includes not only surgical processes but pre-operative, operative and post-operative procedures (those in the clinic, theatre and ward), as well as the activities that support these within the Trust as a whole (presentations at meetings, teaching and learning, setting up new systems, finding out about new ideas). (See Chapter 10.)

Theme 6: Developing

This is about all the professional developments needed and activities engaged in, in order to develop the being, doing, knowing and thinking.

For example, this encompasses all those processes of investigation and research through which the teacher seeks to evaluate the education that has been offered, and the learning practitioner seeks to gain further education. This would include: learning more about career pathways and how to develop within the profession as a whole; learning new techniques and procedures; gaining new knowledge including self-knowledge; working out into the wider professional community; reading research *critically*; writing up and publishing research. We have focused particularly here upon coming to understand practice better through reflection as educational enquiry, which we see as an overarching activity in all the above (see Chapter 11).

We hope that by all these means we have provided readers with a variety of ways of looking at the arguments we offer, and of finding their way to sections they may need to re-read and or use.

We have addressed both the teacher and the learner in this text, since cultivating a thinking surgeon involves both cultivating thinking surgical teachers, and developing pro-active learners. We believe that this book can offer fertile ground for engaging in a learning partnership in the practice setting. We believe that our contribution will be relevant and will provide important perspectives that may otherwise be overlooked, whatever the fate of the various curricula now in development for teaching in the clinical setting.

We would remind readers that education books are not to be read like novels, or treated like a 'work-book', which has to be worked through in page order, but used to pursue and deepen ideas and understanding. We hope this book can be used at the relevant point in practice, when teacher and learner are looking for a challenge to their thinking and activities to take their educational practice further.

This book is no more than a beginning, a contribution to a debate that we hope will ultimately enhance the way that surgeons are prepared for practice. But this will only be so if readers engage critically with what we offer, and reshape or develop it further. In the end, it is not our own ideas that matter, but whether and how the surgical profession can move forward with real progress. Education of a profession, for a profession and by a profession, is an enterprise that is central to its continued health. The survival and development of surgical practice depends upon sound education. We all need it to be successful. We all have a part to play.

Note: Throughout the book we have deliberately used, with reference to surgeons who are receiving postgraduate education as part of their post, both the terms 'trainees' and 'learning surgeons', but with a greater emphasis on the latter. In doing so we believe that we are reflecting the stage that the surgical profession has currently reached in moving gradually away from seeing the enterprise of postgraduate medicine as training and towards seeing it as education.

Linda de Cossart and Della Fish
February 2005

Part one

The educational foundation for cultivating a thinking surgeon

Chapter 1

The significance of clinical practice in the education of a surgeon

Introduction

Traditional ways of teaching and learning in surgery
Traditional National Health Service (NHS) Consultant Surgeons and their role as trainer
Traditional styles of teaching and learning
Learning by apprenticeship
Recent experiences of the learner

The changing world of surgical education and training
The Calman reforms
Modernising Medical Careers
Regulation of the medical profession

From traditional training to new ways of cultivating a surgeon
The context for teaching and learning in modern surgical practice
The nature of clinical practice and what needs to be taught
New styles of teaching and learning
The learner's needs
Clinical practice and learning through reflection in the 21st Century

Introduction

Surgeons have always valued the richness of clinical practice as providing opportunities for teaching. While its educational significance must remain central, the ways of using it for surgical teaching will have to change under the new circumstances of the 21st Century.

In the past the clinical setting was viewed as the arena in which surgeons could demonstrate clinical cases and instruct the learner in clinical and operative procedures. This was eminently possible in the last four decades of the 20th Century when surgeons worked long hours and had significant control of their practice, when each day's worth of clinical practice was worked through until it was completed, when patients spent longer in hospital and when learning surgeons immersed themselves in the activities of practice often to the exclusion of other aspects of life. Surgeons currently in the second and third decades of their consultant careers (and who are today's key teachers in surgery) will be very familiar with this vocational way of life. However, the importance of the more complex aspects of the young surgeons' development such as clinical and professional judgement, were left implicit and thus unexamined.

The educational assumptions beneath this way of training surgeons were that endless repetition of activity in practice was the mainstay of developing and refining it. A lengthy period spent in training was assumed to be important both to develop practical experience and mature its underlying clinical judgement. The assessment of surgeons' practical expertise rested largely on observation of them by those with whom they worked closely and who had significant control over their progress. This was probably more rigorous than it has been given credit for but there was no formal assessment of operative or clinical ability. The old style Fellowship examination of the Royal College of Surgeons (FRCS) (which was in use prior to the current Intercollegiate examination) was taken early in a surgical career. It provided a way into the training pathway rather than an accreditation at the end of training which would indicate expertise gained. Examinations at the end of training programmes in the specialties of surgery have been under development since the early 1990s. Success in them provides evidence for career progression. The profession is still wrestling with refining the process.

We therefore endorse the developing view that in the 21st Century, given the current pressures on ways of working (and therefore also of learning), and the need to develop surgeons at a pace commensurate with the needs of the NHS, the clinical setting must continue to be seen as the fundamental educational resource for teachers and learners. However, the current service environment will require teachers of surgeons to adopt new methods and approaches to education to ensure that the clinical setting maintains this central role. Consultants who teach must come to see themselves as a resource rather than a didactic teacher, and as part of a much wider inter-professional education team, rather than the only surgical educator. It will also require the wider community of the NHS to embrace and support these imperatives. Strong leadership will be essential to its success. The consultant will become the co-ordinator of educational provision and assessment. Learners will need to be far more pro-active in seeking to learn from everyone and everything, and will be responsible for collecting and presenting the evidence of their own learning.

This chapter aims to offer the reader an analysis of each of these ways of engaging in teaching and learning in clinical settings, and thus indicate what is involved in moving from traditional training to new ways of teaching surgeons, and from seeking to produce a skilled technician to striving to cultivate a thinking surgeon.

Traditional ways of teaching and learning in surgery

Traditional NHS Consultant Surgeons and their role as trainer

Traditional NHS consultant surgeons have always seen teaching as part of their professional responsibilities, many committing a large part of their own time and energy to this undertaking.

Few, if any, had time in their job plan to do this. The capable body of surgeons currently joining surgical practice as consultants is a credit to such commitment as well as to their personal experience of an excess of 30,000 hours of clinical work supporting the service requirements of the NHS before consultant appointment (Chickwe, de Souza and Pepper, 2004). Traditional teaching however, has been driven by the need to pass examinations and to improve the curriculum vitae (CV) of the trainee in order to increase their competitiveness at the next round of job interviews. It has produced a practitioner with a very focused view of professional practice, a very career-directed attitude to life, and some disinclination to take on board new ideas about teaching and learning.

The examination syllabus, certainly in the early years of training, has provided the content of teaching sessions, which usually take place in the classroom. These are consultant led and consultant driven, as are ideas for audit and research. They alone have tended to shape the learner's view of what their postgraduate education is about. Examinations, as evidence for capability, have taken more prominence throughout the last ten years because confidence in the profession's assessment of learners' progress and ability has been debased, seen as mere opinion and suspected as open to bias.

Learning to *be* a surgeon, however, and the operative and clinical skills that this requires has always been something to be learned 'on the job'. But strangely, these practical activities, not being presented as classroom lectures, were often not counted as teaching by the learner. Indeed, learning in clinical settings by Senior House Officers (SHOs) has been described as 'opportunistic' and 'magpie-like' without much guidance on the content and the quality of the experience (Brigley *et al*, 2003). This is hardly surprising since opportunities to learn in the clinical setting have become fewer. Parallel operating lists, where the traditional senior/registrar learned to operate as the lead surgeon with a consultant in the adjacent operating theatre were much valued as a teaching resource but are now a long gone phenomenon. This followed a stance taken by the profession (bowing to social concerns about patient safety) to veto them. This view arose from the inability of the profession to demonstrate the evidence for surgeons in training being ready to undertake such independent operating. Sadly, there was never a requirement to replace parallel operating lists with any other scheduled operative teaching opportunities. As a consequence, young surgeons, SHOs in particular, find it difficult to gain opportunities to learn and develop their operative skills in the clinical setting (de Cossart, Wiltshire and Brown, 2001; Katory, Singh and Beard, 2001). Recent moves to prepare senior nurses and other advanced practitioners to work as first assistants in theatre or to become surgical care practitioners, are also decreasing the opportunities of surgical SHOs to gain practical experience. Ironically, this is further compounded by the need for consultants to spend more time teaching operative surgery to an increasingly inexperienced generation of registrars in higher surgical training, and by the service requirement for SHOs to manage the wards.

The sessions freed up by the 1995 decision have now been swallowed up by service demands, which have ignored the need for operative teaching. Managers and all those who have educational responsibility for the profession need to recognize that this will lead to an increasingly disabled surgical workforce. Provision for learning operative procedures urgently needs to be put in place.

At the same time as these problems were emerging, both simulation exercises and master classes were being developed. It was believed by some that they would not only supplement theoretical teaching but also would compensate for shortfalls in operative teaching and learning in the clinical setting. Great expertise in simulation now provides innovative ways of instructing, practising and honing such skills. They do not however, simulate the real operating room environment with its unpredictable complexities and individual patient needs.

It is hardly surprising therefore, that up to now traditional teaching in surgery has been increasingly focused on that which can be offered in the classroom and in skills facilities.

Figure 1:1 shows the essence of this view of 'training' a surgeon. It indicates that formal education for the postgraduate doctor is conceived as a matter of the surgical teacher taking the responsibility of providing and preparing the content and formally instructing the learner, who attends, receives and absorbs. Such education is seen as formal teaching in the classroom setting (often in the postgraduate medical centre, well away from the clinical setting), and is intended to prepare candidates for the examination process, thus focusing upon theoretical knowledge and changing patterns of behaviour in the trainee in order to improve their chances of passing the exam. Little if any time is devoted to exploring the understanding that the learner develops either from these classroom sessions or from clinical practice. In particular, the effect on their subsequent ability to work as a surgeon in the clinical setting is rarely explored.

By contrast, training the surgeon in practical skills is seen as coaching, and takes place in the clinical setting in ward, theatre and clinic, but when and only when service and time permit. This is because 'coaching' here tends to mean the learner working under the direct instruction of the surgical teacher, at a high level of supervision, which slows down the procedure being taught and the Trust through-put, makes learners teacher-dependent, and does not empower them to move quickly to higher levels of practice. Further, learners in this mode of teaching get little support in recognizing how they learn, in developing their understanding, or knowing whether they are progressing satisfactorily. Reflecting on and recording their development is non-existent. In fact, apart from a log of operative procedures and a list of courses attended, there is no requirement to produce a meaningful record of their range of competence. This means that there is no process to demonstrate competence to undertake operations and manage patients, and no evidence of this to be shared with managers or patients. In learning in the clinical setting, quantity has always been a measure of surgical development. This has led to high value being placed by both teacher and learner on doing large numbers of operations. This mindset is bound for disaster in the current climate of change in the NHS.

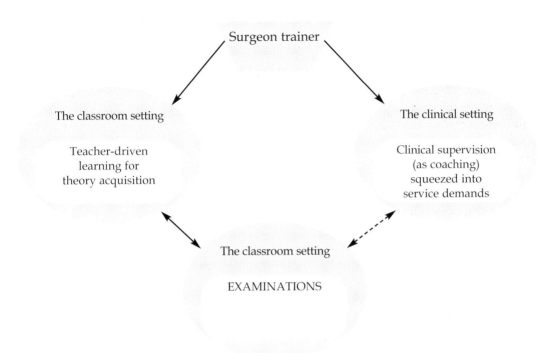

Figure 1:1 Traditional NHS surgeons in their role as trainers.

Traditional styles of teaching and learning

The style of teaching (and by default therefore learning) in this traditional view can be characterized as follows.

- Teacher is the 'Authority', and hierarchical relationships govern all teaching interactions.
- It is exam driven.
- The aim of teacher and learner is to improve learners' CVs in order to increase competitiveness in gaining the next job.
- The educational aim assumes that theory should be taught and then *applied* to practice.
- Such teaching values measurable achievement (numbers of exams and rate of achievement, Doctors of Medicine (MD) and Masters of Surgery (MS)).
- Teacher and learner both value high numbers of procedures/operations carried out.
- Teachers and learners most value the acquisition of advanced surgical skills, seeing routine procedures and other professional attributes as inferior.
- There is little if any structured clinical assessment.

Endemic to the above view of training a surgeon, has been the conviction that any teaching and learning in the clinical setting is about 'learning by apprenticeship'. Traditional consultant surgeons believe that the loss of this form of teaching, as a consequence of new ways of working imposed by the European Working Time Directive (EWTD), will be disastrous. But these new demands, as we shall show, provide an opportunity to develop new ways of teaching in clinical settings. However, we should first explore what surgeons mean and understand by apprenticeship, and what they believe it involves, and ask whether they have actually critiqued the notion that they automatically support.

Learning by apprenticeship

It is probably fair to say that the term 'apprenticeship' is used uncritically by surgeons as a shorthand (but rather inaccurate) way of referring to the teaching that goes on in clinical settings. Macdonald noted that the literature shows that 'in spite of the ubiquity of the concept and the high value placed on apprenticeship by the medical profession, neither a great deal of information, nor in-depth descriptions are available to clarify how apprenticeship takes place', (Macdonald, 1997, p. 11). The general sense that apprenticeship is what surgeons offer young doctors, is probably more apparent than real, and certainly there have been few attempts to explore it (the articles by Buckley, 1995; and Bleakley, 2002; being among the few exceptions). The sense that medical education is a form of apprenticeship has no doubt developed because learning surgery seems (on the surface) very like the traditional tradesman's apprenticeship. Both types of teaching and learning are carried out in the practical setting; the content to be taught is seen as 'skills'; the means of teaching is talking and demonstrating; the way of learning is to listen and to apply exactly in practice what the teacher has shown and taught; the teacher is a kind of 'master'; the learner is placed with the teacher in the teacher's natural setting for their work; the learner is in lower level employment, alongside the teacher, for a set period of time; there is an end assessment which acts as a gateway into further practice. Because they have seen surgery largely as a craft specialty, surgeons have readily empathized with this description of the way they work, teach and learn.

However, we would argue that of far more significance than the similarities between craft apprentices and surgeons are some deep and serious differences, which emerge in a closer and more detailed scrutiny of apprenticeship. For example, The Oxford English Dictionary (OED) provides the following details of origin and definition. The Prentice, or Apprentice first appears in Middle English (14th Century) as: 'one who is a learner of a craft; one who is bound by a legal agreement to serve an employer for a period of seven years with a view to learning some handicraft or trade, in which the employer is reciprocally bound to instruct him.' (OED.) Modern dictionaries demonstrate that the term has not lost this early association, defining an apprentice as 'one bound to another to learn a craft, a mere novice'; and offering for apprenticeship: 'a term of practical training still referred to as seven years'. (Chambers Dictionary.) Apprenticeship was thus a fair term for the early barber surgeons who were without medical qualifications.

Since the 14th Century, then, the term apprenticeship has been used in the context of the production of craft and handicraft workers, for whom training (instruction in, and the exercise of) essential skills was the entire and sufficient educational activity. Such workers, of course, were part of the industrial production process and were concerned with the making of objects. They were usually school leavers who were deemed suitable to learn practical skills without serious theoretical foundations. Their learning was not in the context of higher education. They were seeking to join a trade or craft. They were not expected to see their role in any wider form of service to the public, nor to their country. The traditions of their practice were relatively simple. They had a fixed job plan and would never expect wide autonomy in their work. Their task was to learn skills, and to emerge at the end with a clear set number of these. By that stage they would not be expecting to have to learn anything further in a formal teaching/learning setting. They would not become graduates and there would be no long-term professional development. They would not expect, during their careers, to extend their abilities to new and more complex jobs.

The learners' role during their apprenticeship was to model the master. This involved learning practical processes (without associated complex theoretical knowledge), and applying these, exactly, (to inert objects), without deviation, and thus achieving the same end product on every occasion. Further, apprenticeship has at base a particular view of the processes of teaching and learning. Here, teaching provides (for a clearly defined and relatively short period) some clear-cut instruction and demonstration and the learner puts this practical knowledge into operation, by following the teacher's processes as precisely as possible. During this process, practical knowledge is applied (to an object), with a view to the replication of process and end. Further, there is not expected to be any new knowledge created during that practical process. It is valid to describe this interaction in terms of 'training'.

By contrast, the modern professional surgeon, who is both a physician and an artist (rather than a craftsman), draws upon complex theoretical knowledge, together with professional judgement, in order to tailor *general* clinical knowledge to the practical treatment of the individual patient's *particular* case. Here, neither the processes nor the end product can be described as exactly the same on every occasion. Rather, they are particular and even unique. What is more, the professional engages in a life-long process of professional development during which a wide range of teaching and learning processes are drawn upon. Here it is necessary to continue, throughout the professional's career, to learn a wide and complex range of both theoretical and practical knowledge. During this process the professional is learning to go beyond what he/she has been taught and to create - during practice - new knowledge in response to ever-new particular and unique human situations. Such learning is a necessary preparation for the complex actions and fine judgements which professionals make with, and on behalf of, human beings.

In the light of this critique, surgeons would do well to consider the appropriateness to their education of the term apprenticeship and whether it is a sufficiently accurate way of characterizing how surgeons should be developed. This is especially so if they are to engage with others, such as educationists, managers, politicians and other members of the multi-disciplinary workforce in medicine, who will in the future be highly influential in the development of postgraduate medical education, and who may bring with them their own ideas of how to reshape teaching and learning in surgery. They may wish to attend mainly to the skills (competencies) element of surgery and as a result fail to recognize the more demanding need to develop competent surgeons who are holistic in their patient care and who exercise fine judgement.

Table 1:1 A summary of the crucial differences between the craft apprentice and the learning surgeon.

The craft apprentice:	The learning surgeon:
• does not usually have a university degree	• always has a university degree (5 years in undergraduate education)
• is usually in their first job after leaving school	• will have done a pre-registration year and will be in anything from year 2 to year 12 after medical school
• will not have any autonomy in their work	• will have a proportion of autonomy and will at times work independently within their experience
• will have a fixed job plan	• will not have a very tightly described job plan
• will have a skills based training programme	• will have a range of educational needs well beyond the skills part of the practice
• will not be bound by any professional tradition in their future jobs	• will be bound by their professional history and the traditions of their practice
• will have a set number of skills and abilities at the end of their apprenticeship	• will have a wide-ranging skills ability at the end of their education and training
• will not usually be involved in post-apprenticeship skills development	• will always be involved in post-accreditation development
• is not in postgraduate education	• is in postgraduate education
• is not in higher education	• is in higher education
• may not have a nationally agreed qualification	• will always have a nationally (and sometimes an internationally) acceptable qualification
• will not necessarily see their role in the wider context of society	• will (or at least should) see their role in the wider context of society and the profession
• is not expected to use discretion	• uses discretion centrally in his or her work
• will not usually have demands made on him or her outside a specific job or skilled performance	• always has demands on him or her outside the undertaking of a specific operation or procedure
• needs practical knowledge	• needs a wide range of knowledge (see Chapter 9)
• creates and works on objects	• works on and with human beings and is involved with life and death decisions

How then do learners see their education now, at a time when old traditions are being challenged and new approaches forecast?

Recent experiences of the learner

Investigation into how surgeons learn in clinical practice at the very beginning of the 21st Century has largely consisted of investigating what formal teaching sessions young surgeons receive along with the number of operations that they are able to perform (Katory, Singh and Beard, 2001). In 2003, more revealing information was gleaned from the research commissioned by the Royal College of Surgeons of England (RCS Eng) as part of its need to evaluate the ideas expressed in the new values-based curriculum of surgical education called 'The Curriculum for the General Professional Practice of Surgery' (GPPS). (See RCS Eng, 2003).

The findings reported by this study describe the general experiences of SHOs and their consultant trainers, based on a carefully designed process of interview and observation. The feelings expressed by SHOs in surgery are consonant with those of their consultants in believing that despite surgery being a craft specialty with the technical aspects being a highly valued part of the practice, being a good surgeon is far more than 'hands on' performance. The study showed that even in the 21st Century an authoritarian style of teaching exists, with SHOs often reluctant to question the authority of the consultant. The hierarchical structure that places consultants at the top and learners below them is prevalent; the consultant telling and the learner 'absorbing' is expected; and some consultants were seemingly oblivious of whether their learners were actually understanding what they were being offered. The attaining of success in examinations, as part of the culture of testing, is seen as the main hurdle to allow progress. There is no rigorous assessment of clinical capability. The concept of reflective practice as a method of teaching and learning is virtually unknown. With the increasing self-assuredness of the modern generation of young people, this attitude of the profession in general will need to change to ensure that young doctors are not discouraged from being keen to make a career in surgery. Amongst SHOs there is a very real feeling that there is no time to teach them and that service needs take precedence over their training.

A supportive and caring department of surgery and a nurturing teaching environment are seen as the most conducive context in which to learn. Successful departments, both clinically and educationally, are those with an ethos of mutual support and development of members, including trainees. They are learning communities. This success is largely founded on the commitment and determination of individual members rather than on the physical facilities provided.

In the light of these issues we must ask how surgical education has come to be where it is at the beginning of the 21st Century.

The changing world of surgical education and training

The Calman reforms

In 1993, Sir Kenneth Calman introduced reforms for specialist registrar training to align the United Kingdom (UK) with the European Union Directive on medical training. The career-training pathway that has evolved as a consequence of this is shown in Figure 1.2. It was envisaged that along with this shorter time-based training there would develop better-structured learning opportunities, supervision and assessment. Despite this intention, training times in most surgical specialties have not shortened and still remain at about twelve years from qualification. This is largely due to the need to spend five or more years in the SHO grade before beginning specialist registrar training. The quality of educational development which would enhance the education of young surgeons has been slow to evolve.

In 1998, the EWTD became part of British law and this is now restricting the time that surgeons may lawfully work. Indeed, there will soon come a time when no doctor will be allowed to work more than 48 hours a week. It is estimated that the effect of this will be to reduce the thirty thousand hours of clinical experience of previously appointed consultants to a mere six thousand (Chickwe, de Souza and Pepper, 2004).

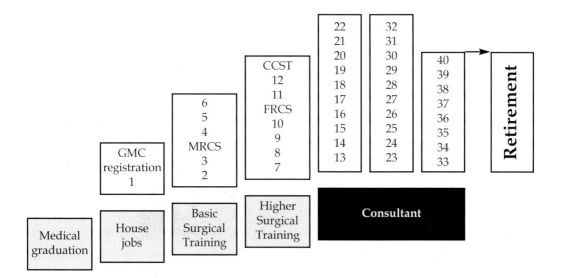

Figure 1: 2 The surgical career pathway for the late 20th Century (numbers indicate years after graduation). *Assumes 40 years in employment (however, the average age of retirement is 58 years); graduation at 24 years; and retirement at 65 years.*

Modernising Medical Careers

The early 21st Century initiatives from the Department of Health (DoH), enshrined in *Modernising Medical Careers* and *A Firm Foundation*, showed DoH ambitions further to reform medical education and training with the determined aim to shorten the time between entry to medical school and acquisition of a Certificate of Completion of Training (CCT) (see Figure 1:3). Newly graduated doctors are about to be required to undertake a compulsory two years of generic clinical work (Foundation Year one and two (F1 and F2)), designed to expose them to a wide range of clinical practice and ensure that they are able to recognize and initiate management of the acutely sick patient. To qualify for a CCT will take between four to six years, and will result in a generalist who is able to work within a defined clinical framework. As this book goes to press, however, discussion is taking place about the establishment of one extra year, to follow the Foundation Programme, which will precede specialist training in some surgical specialties.

In addition to this, some generalists will progress and develop further to obtain a Certificate of Completion of Specialist Training (CCST). How precisely this will happen is unclear and will no doubt evolve. It is envisaged that some generalist consultants will, as a planned programme within their consultant job, develop further specialised areas of their practice (see Figure 1:3).

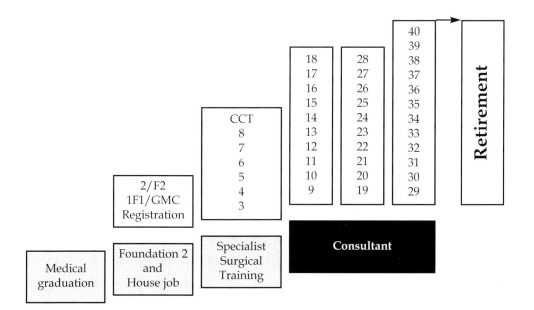

Figure 1:3 The proposed surgical career pathway for the 21st Century (numbers indicate years after graduation). *Assumes 40 years in employment; graduation at 24 years; and retirement at 65 years. The place of the CCST is as yet uncertain but is proposed at some time during consultant appointment.*

Regulation of the medical profession

Teachers in surgical practice are now expected to maintain the standard set by the General Medical Council (GMC) in *Good Medical Practice* (2001) which states: 'if you have responsibilities for teaching you must develop the skills, attitudes and practices of a competent teacher.' (GMC, 2001). The challenge for surgical teachers is to provide for the development of new surgeons with few of the resources they need to do this and in a shorter period of time. We believe that the curriculum for each phase of this new process will need to be refined over at least the next decade.

The regulation of standards and evidence for practice is now a requirement by Trust processes for clinical governance. Appraisal, the Clinical Negligence Schemes for Trusts, along with the new Postgraduate Medical Education and Training Board (PMETB), will demand clear standards and demonstration of those standards by all involved in service and educational practice in the NHS. This is a tall order, and is being introduced at great speed and in the context of many other sweeping innovations like appraisal, revalidation and the new consultant contract.

Highly motivated trainees and consultant teachers will be thoroughly demoralised if they do not take stock of their position in this changing world. Reconstructing ideas about surgical teaching will need both surgical and teaching expertise if the standards of surgical practice currently enjoyed by society are to be maintained, let alone developed. This will only happen if teaching and learning is given status and is not regarded as the hobby of an enthusiast. Teaching must be seen to be as important as service delivery. Visionary surgeons and educationists who are able to see beyond the apparent stranglehold of the present situation must think clearly and strategically in order to make this happen. Only surgeons know what it takes to be a good surgeon; only teachers know what it takes to be a good teacher. Only by combining the expertise of these two professions in those who teach surgeons in the future will we safeguard the standards of surgical education.

From traditional training to new ways of cultivating a surgeon

The richness of surgical practice will not change. How surgeons see themselves in the role of surgical teacher must however change as a consequence of the reforms. It is likely that in the future not all consultants will play a significant part in teaching. Those who choose to take on such a role must first ensure that they understand the responsibility they are assuming. They must have a clear idea of the type of practitioner (technician or professional) that they wish to be involved in developing. We believe that if surgeons are to be doctors with professional responsibilities in addition to being skilled technicians, their teachers will need to attend to a wide-ranging curriculum (as well as to the development of surgical skills), and especially to the issue of professional judgement. Surgeons will need to refine their development as teachers and educators. They will need to believe in themselves as surgical teachers but respect from others will need to be earned. They will need to be able to make the case for cultivating the type of surgeon who can respond fully to the humanistic and surgical needs of patients.

The context for teaching and learning in modern surgical practice

The clinical setting enables learners to find ways of seeing, and importantly, exploring and understanding the complexities of surgical practice. It is the right arena in which to develop ways of seeing and attending to holistic patient care and learner-centred education. It will allow the observation, investigation and critique of real examples of professional judgement in both medical and educational practice, by both teacher and learner. It will allow creative thinking and safe improvisation and the valuing and development of self-knowledge and self-appraisal. In all this, the surgical teacher will be the ever-visible model for the learner, and will need to establish a safe learning environment for learner and patient.

The clinical setting provides endless opportunity for the teacher to utilize a range of ways of engaging learners in relevant practical activities, which will develop their problem-solving capabilities. It also provides the opportunity to encourage and model many other things including critical thinking (as a cast of mind and way of thinking); the ability to engage in deliberation; and the valuing of reflection, by demonstrating and making time for this important way of enabling learners to clarify and solidify their learning. All consultants engage each day in familiar and habitual activities, which have become subconscious over the years and are interpreted by observers as an intuitive (but puzzling) reaction to a situation. Teachers will need to make overt their tacit knowledge involved, which otherwise will be unclear and unstated to learners. Failing to do this will slow down the learners' development.

The good teacher therefore, is one who ensures that they themselves are capable of using the clinical setting for these important opportunities, which must, in turn, be valued by the wider surgical profession and by those who manage and run the NHS.

The nature of clinical practice and what needs to be taught

Clinical practice involves surgeons engaging with people who are ill and negotiating with them a plan of care appropriate to their needs and wants. Patients want and expect an honest and empathetic response from their surgeon, whom they see as an expert and in a position to help them. They want to be given time, and be treated with dignity and as a fellow human being. They value being part of the decision-making process, as shown by Britton (2004).

The surgeon, the patient and their loved ones all bring to the consultation expectations, values and feelings, which will influence their reactions to what happens. Surgeons need to be able to call on a depth of specific knowledge to be able to advise appropriately. In a discipline where changes are happening all the time and where communication is faster than ever before, this is a big task. The surgeon must be able to take a salient history, perform an examination, investigate, diagnose, and come to a clinical solution (which may or may not include an operation). A process of deliberation with the patient must then turn this into an agreed plan of treatment. The surgeon's role here is to guide the patient in the best way of managing their problem from their point of view. The measure of success of the consultation between patient and surgeon will depend on the patient's perception of whether or not the surgeon has offered them what they want to know, and treated them with respect and appropriate surgical expertise. It is perhaps salutary to reflect that sometimes even when things do not go as planned, if the patient feels that they have been given respect by their surgeon, they still express gratitude and thanks. Patients understand that doctors cannot perform miracles, but it does need the surgeon to realise this too.

During this process of consultation and treatment, a wide range of people with whom the surgeon works will observe, and have their own values, beliefs and opinions about the conduct of all involved in the consultation and its outcome. The surgeon works in a complex and even messy environment where things are rarely the same twice. Experience builds up trends of successful and unsuccessful ways of doing things. But, as well as responding to these human interactions and possessing a great depth of factual knowledge, surgeons needs to understand their own position with respect to their technical and operative ability. They must work to the standards set down by their profession. They need also to know the requirements of the organization in which they work and its appropriateness for providing safely the treatment to be offered. Learning doctors working in this complex and messy environment need to be guided to develop insight into how to think as well as ways of coping with a very demanding environment.

Figure 1:4 indicates the range of knowledge that is therefore needed to develop a surgeon. It indicates that all teaching and learning in postgraduate medicine in future will need to take place in the clinical setting, or in rooms nearby. It raises the status of education as equal in importance to service.

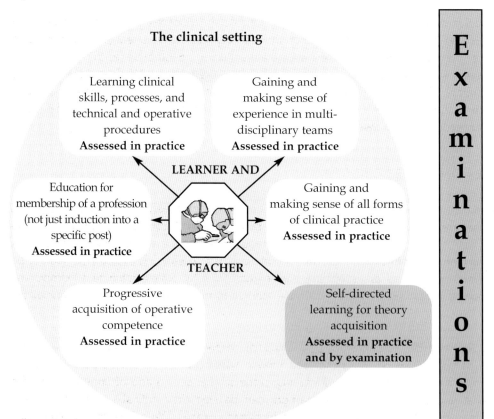

Figure 1:4 Teaching and learning for surgical practice.

New styles of teaching and learning

The following characterizes the new approaches to the education of surgeons. It will involve:

- a wider range of activities in teaching and learning;
- a learner-centred approach with learners taking responsibility for documenting the evidence of their development;
- the use of reflective practice to enhance understanding of and draw wisdom from experience gained;
- seeing theory as necessary for practice but recognizing that new theories can be generated in practice;
- new ways of motivating learners and teachers;
- valuing specificity about which operational procedures the learner has become successful in;
- valuing preparing the learner for belonging to a profession;
- recognizing that while learning on the attachment, the learner is part of a larger community of practice;
- assessing all elements in the practice setting with a rigour that also ensures they are recorded in the learning portfolio.

The clinical setting offers the best and most appropriate educational resource to provide for this as well as the opportunities to assess the learning surgeon in a real life environment. It facilitates the involvement of relevant multi-disciplinary contributions to learning and assessment, which will enrich a young surgeon's development. Working in the clinical environment is what surgeons like doing because it is the heart of surgical practice. It is why they went to medical school. It is the backdrop for their continuing development. Therefore, there is no better place to foster the learning of the professional practice of surgery.

The learner's needs

Learning in the clinical environment needs to be seen by both learner and teacher as part of and not separate from service. All events must be seen as both clinical and educational. The learning that can occur here needs to be recognized as the norm. The main form of communication during this exchange will be oral, and these exchanges themselves need to be explored and considered systematically and learned from by both teacher and learner. The importance of these opportunities is for the learner to make their own meaning out of the teaching they have been given.

Protected surgical teaching time is essential, especially for learning operative skills. However, it should not be restricted to a narrow surgical focus. It must also be used for developing the generic principles of learning in the clinical setting and of understanding the educational methods through which learners can develop their criticality, scepticism, self-directed learning, reflective practice and an educational portfolio. We believe that on the whole, in current surgical practice, no time at all is given over to these aspects of a trainee's development, but that doing so in future will make a huge difference to the amount of value gained from the teaching/learning interaction. Surgeons need to respond to a wide range of scenarios in their clinical practice and in all of them they are expected to act appropriately. Learning must therefore be directed to the development of the qualities espoused on becoming a member of a profession, including the acquisition of the capacity for sound judgement, together with flexibility and a variety of interpersonal skills and attributes.

Clinical practice and learning through reflection in the 21st Century

Surgical work in the future, then, will need to combine both clinical and educational practice to ensure that every opportunity is taken to develop the capacity of the learner during every clinical event. Thus patient-centred and learner-centred interactions will occur at the same time. But having the clinical experience *without* systematic reflection upon it, is to miss much of its importance and meaning. This will require all those who teach young surgeons to provide the time and opportunity to help learners to turn their lived experience into learning as soon as possible.

In other health care professions (for example nursing and physiotherapy) the term used for this overall educational activity (support during the experience and facilitation of the reflection) is 'clinical supervision'. The key roles it is seen to play in many professions are the clinical governance role for the safety of patients, the educational role, and the therapeutic role (which is important for the learner's own well being) (see Proctor, 1986). Of these, we see education as by far the most important (see Fish, 2005). Both the terms 'reflective practice' and 'clinical supervision' provide important language in which to explore modern ways of educating clinicians and also open up the possibilities of learning from the literature of other professions. They are explored in more detail in later chapters of this book.

The above requires an explicit recognition of the professional values which young surgeons need to develop, and the educational values which their teachers need to enact. Accordingly, the next two chapters will deal with these issues and principles.

Chapter 2

Professional values and the traditions of practice in surgery

Introduction

What we mean by professional values and their importance in surgical education

Further explorations of professional values

The use and significance of professional values in teaching and learning in clinical settings

Introduction

Education (like medicine) is not a science which seeks to discover clear and unequivocal answers that are proved, objective, absolute and universal. Like all professional practice, education is founded upon, and begins with, values. These complicate professional education and clinical practice, rendering it problematic, because there will be few universally agreed absolute and final solutions to educational and surgical questions. In surgical education, the first question that must be asked is: what kind of surgeon are we seeking to develop? There are, and always will be, tensions about this matter. Different values and priorities will result in differences of emphasis on technical skills and/or wider capabilities, and the right to offer an answer to this question belongs to many different people and institutions. In their professional work too (from the very beginning and throughout their careers) surgeons are driven by their own complex values and are at the centre of conflicting expectations and requirements of many other people. These all stem from different ways of thinking about what matters most about a surgeon and surgery. For this reason, throughout surgical education, discussion of values with the learning surgeon can provide an important reminder of the fundamental driving forces of professional practice, and an understanding of the root of many practical difficulties.

Without an awareness that this is so, the surgeon and the surgeon educator will experience irritations, but not have the means to grapple with them. It is the responsibility of all surgical teachers to enable young surgeons to explore their own professional values (which arise from their own autobiographies and are made visible daily in the way they conduct themselves). For example, they need to help them consider how their own values relate to those: required of them by their College and the GMC; expected by their teachers, peers and other health care colleagues; looked for by managers, patients and the public; and that are influenced by legal pressures. Turning to values and how they shape all our actions, can also help surgical teachers to talk to the difficult young surgeon whose conduct is unacceptable.

By raising this very matter we are beginning to reveal our own position on values, which is well expressed by Golby, when he says that he thinks of professionals as: 'persons who seek a broad understanding of their practice, paying attention not only to their developing

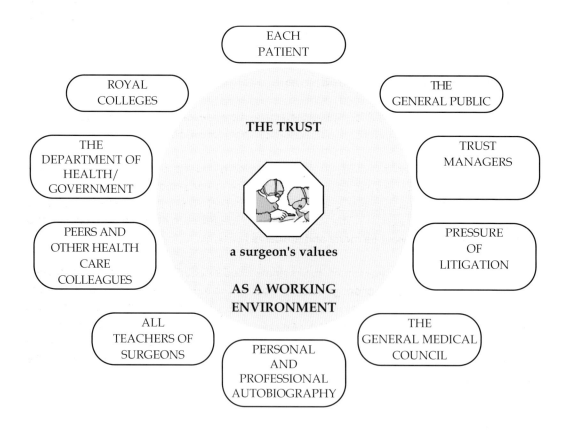

Figure 2:1 Factors influencing the surgeon's values and consequent conduct.

competence, but also to the fundamental purposes and values that underpin their work' (Golby, 1993, p. 5). Readers need to be aware of this as they think critically about what we present and how we present it, not only in this chapter, but throughout the book.

Figure 2:1 illustrates the variety of people and places whose values come to bear on the conduct of surgery. At different times in the surgeon's work, the priority of the various influences will change, but they will always all be present. The educational values which shape the educational approach in surgical settings are discussed in Chapter 3.

This chapter explores, in three sections, values and their fundamental importance for the education of surgeons. The first seeks to define and clarify what is meant by values, the second explores the issues involved in more detail and provides examples, and the third shows the responsibilities that this creates for the teacher and the learner.

What we mean by professional values and their importance in surgical education

This section considers values firstly in relation to the individual professional practitioner; secondly in terms of the responsibilities of a whole profession; and finally in relation to the profession of surgery and the development of surgical education.

Professional values and the individual

Values are those abiding and long-cherished views which we all have as individuals - but do not necessarily share - about what counts as enduringly worthwhile and important.

Our professional values determine how we consistently see the world in which we engage in professional practice. They shape what we prioritize in our professional life and how we conduct ourselves in both clinical and educational settings. That conduct reveals our values to colleagues, patients and learners. The term 'conduct' here refers to the acknowledgement that beneath our visible behaviour lie moral and ethical dimensions.

We subscribe to Hoyle's models of 'the restricted and extended professional', which were first offered in the context of schoolteacher development in a decade in which major changes were being demanded of teachers. In Table 2:1 we have summarised (and slightly adapted in reference to surgery) the characteristics he ascribes in his article to these two different kinds of professional. We believe that this demonstrates the negative model offered to learners by restricted professionals, and illustrates the problems that they will have in responding to the needs of rapidly changing times.

Table 2:1 The restricted and extended professional surgeon (following Hoyle, 1974).

Restricted professional	Extended professional
Own clinical skills are derived from experience	Own clinical skills derived from the mediation between experience and theory of all kinds, through rigorous reflection
Perspectives restricted to 'what happens now' (only short-term goals are of concern)	Perspectives embrace wider social context and later times (long as well as short-term goals are of concern)
Sees clinical practice as technical procedures which merit little educational interest because learning them only requires plenty of repetition	Sees clinical practice as complex, intriguing, problematic, driven by values, beliefs, assumptions and needing to be seated in a professional philosophy
Clinical events are seen in isolation each from the other and from any wider perspectives	Clinical events seen in relation to social policies and wider goals
Introspective about own clinical methods and processes	Clinical methods and processes compared with colleagues and with reports of other practice
High value placed on own autonomy	Value placed on professional collaboration within and beyond own profession
Limited involvement in all but direct clinical activities	High value on the whole range of professional activities - locally, within Trust, and nationally
Infrequent reading of a range of literature beyond immediate clinical specialty	Frequent reading of a wide range of literature relevant to professional practice generally
Least possible involvement in professional development (and only at personal level)	Involvement in professional development at a range of levels (personal and collegiate)
Sees no personal gain in teaching younger colleagues	Recognizes range of reasons to engage in the education of fellow professionals

Values, then, are a form of motivation which underlies behaviour. They are held consistently, and their moral seriousness should be able to be justified. They are the established currencies in things about which people care. They are shaped in us by our education, experience and cultural heritage.

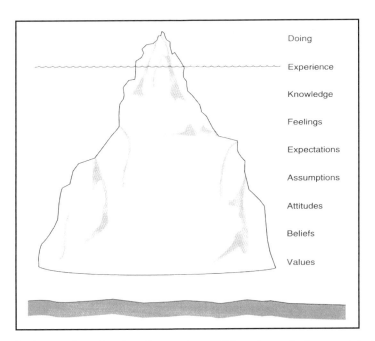

Doing

Experience

Knowledge

Feelings

Expectations

Assumptions

Attitudes

Beliefs

Values

Figure 2:2 The iceberg of professional practice. With acknowledgement to the work of Fish and Coles, 1998.

Values thus drive our actions, attitudes, thoughts and beliefs. Their central role in professional practice in both medicine and education is illustrated by Fish and Coles in Figure 2:2 in which they characterize professional practice as an iceberg. The visible performance of the professional (a very small proportion of the whole) is underpinned by a range of invisible but highly significant tacit resources and underlying drives, the foundation of which is values.

Espoused values and values-in-use

Espoused values are those values we put into *words* when asked what we believe. They are discernible beneath what we say we would do if we had a choice about our professional conduct. By contrast, our values-in-use are revealed through our *actions*. Actions speak louder than words. It is in our actions that people see what we really believe. Whilst our espoused values and our values-in-use are in harmony, there is no conflict, but this is rare, and something to strive for, rather than something we can easily attain.

However, conflict frequently arises from two sorts of problems. It arises on the one hand where an individual is restrained by other values systems from doing what he believes in, and is required to find a suitable compromise. On the other hand, it occurs where an individual says one thing (because it appears the right or popular thing to say) but freely acts in a different way.

When we recognize such conflict, it is important to explore both our practice and our values further. When we do so we may discover values that we should act upon but which we have not prioritized and which therefore may be lost. A key example of this would be the failure to prioritize educational activities in the light of a target-driven culture, where one view of what professional practice is about (i.e. the rapid through-put of patients) blinkers its proponents to any other view, and (we would argue) is threatening the quality of both education and health care. Alternatively, we may sometimes have to concede that our espoused values are unable to be achieved in the current situation, that the case to prioritize them has not been made, that we need to find a compromise position, or that they are truly inappropriate. (But we do not think that this is true of the above example - even in the short term.)

The values of a profession

Every profession works on the basis of profession-wide values, whether tacit or declared.

The clarification, written statement and regular updating of a profession's values is vital in a number of ways. It:

- ❑ provides the public and professional regulators with explicit parameters of professional conduct, which can be currently expected of members of that profession;
- ❑ provides educators of new entrants to the profession with the basis for helping them to recognize, and scrutinize critically the values of the profession they are joining;
- ❑ provides intending entrants to the profession with a basis from which to consider their own values and the relationship of these to those of the profession;
- ❑ provides teachers, learners, assessors, evaluators and the profession with one starting point for the rationale for professional education;
- ❑ provides curriculum developers with a proper basis for ensuring that all the key elements of the curriculum fully support the values of the profession and the consequent needs of learners;
- ❑ provides examiners and assessors with the basis for deciding the purposes of assessment, what should be assessed, and how;
- ❑ provides all relevant parties with a properly explicit basis for review, critique, and development of the curriculum itself.

Public statements about values (personal or institutional) meet the following standards. They: are chosen from alternatives; enhance conduct and our ability to explain and defend it; are consistent with each other; should be easily communicable; should be limited in number; should give pride to the enterprise; should be genuinely actionable; should be written down; and should be able to be lived.

The values of any profession emerge over time and have in common the fact that:

- ❑ they have historical roots;
- ❑ they grow out of an understanding of what is involved in being a particular kind of professional practitioner;

❏   they are influenced by the developing traditions of professional practice;

❏   they recognize the values of the current context within which that practice is taking place.

Members of a number of health care professions have recently explored the significance of their professionalism (Davies, 1998; Saks, 1998; and Fish and Coles, 1998), and some have asked whether professionalism is coming to an end (Southern and Braithwaite, 1998; Pereira Grey, 2002). But it is Freidson who has shown us how to nurture and develop professionalism in the current climate (Freidson, 1994 and 2001), and O'Neill, who argues the importance of preserving trust between patients and professionals, and the danger of eroding professionalism in the current attitudes of the media and the public (O'Neill, 2002).

Surgical values

The profession of surgery has not until now set down its values for clear public scrutiny, although they have been implicit in acceptable surgical practice. They are currently being formulated through new developments in the surgical curriculum. The following illustrates some of the key influences on their development.

The historical roots for surgeons' professional values

An early statement of the values of which the Royal College of Surgeons of England declared itself the guardian, appeared thus in its Charter in 1800:

'... the object of the College is the promotion of the art and science of surgery and the promotion and encouragement of the study and practice of the said art and science.'

(RCS Eng, 1996)

The importance to surgeons of both scientific knowledge and procedures, and of the aspects of their practice which are less easily defined (the professional artistry of practice), are highlighted in this statement. It also calls for the nurturing of learning, which inevitably underpins good practice. It remains as relevant in the 21st Century as when it was first written.

Membership of the surgical profession

Surgeons require special courage and confidence in order to be able to operate on patients. They need to have the capacity to cope with the risks and possible complications of their surgery and to respond to the demands for accountability for their technical performance and answerability for the moral and ethical dimensions. For surgeons, membership of their profession means engaging with patients, on whom they perform an overt and calculated injury, before treatment is complete. Their patients will see them as a key thread through their surgical care. The fiduciary relationship of the surgeon with the patient involves special trust in the judgment of the professional, and the surgeon must honour that trust. Their involvement in this complex and discretionary work will require them to have an ethical basis for their actions which brings with it a moral duty.

The current developing traditions of surgical practice

Surgery is a constantly changing practice, which will require surgeons in the 21st Century to respond as never before to new ways of thought and action in their clinical and operative practice. Surgeons' professional responsibilities will demand that they value these developments positively and ensure that they are suitably prepared to meet them. The Royal College of Surgeons' *Good Surgical Practice* (September 2002) acts as a reference point for how surgeons should currently conduct themselves (see RCS Eng, 2002).

The values of the wider medical and social context

In response to the concerns of the public and government about quality, and the prevailing concerns in society about the accountability of members of professions, The General Medical Council has set out standards for all doctors in *Good Medical Practice* (May 2001). This important document requires all doctors to value good standards of practice as described. It:

- ☐ defines good clinical care and its processes;
- ☐ makes explicit expectations about clinical judgement and patients' rights to be treated even if they pose a risk to the doctor;
- ☐ establishes the need to maintain good medical practice and performance;
- ☐ sets standards of objectivity and honesty and requires sound evidence in the assessment of doctors;
- ☐ expects all who teach to be able to demonstrate evidence of being a competent teacher;
- ☐ sets out the conditions for good relationships with patients (consent, trust, confidentiality, communication, ending relationships);
- ☐ provides procedures for dealing with the poor conduct or performance of colleagues;
- ☐ clarifies the expectations for working well with colleagues (treating them fairly);
- ☐ recognizes the importance of working well in teams, leading teams, arranging cover, taking up appointments, sharing information with colleagues, delegation and referral;
- ☐ shapes the minimum requirements for probity (honest information, not pressurizing patients, writing reliable reports);
- ☐ requires the protection of patients' care and safety as a first priority in any research conducted.

(See GMC, 2001)

The importance of professional values in surgical education

Since professional values so profoundly influence the conduct of surgeons in their everyday lives, surgical teachers must be able to explore with learners their own values, their profession's and the relationship between the two. This will allow the learner to do the same. It will also encourage the recognition of values held in common with other health care professionals, thus allowing a common currency by which the care of patients and relationships with colleagues may be shaped.

In the current context, those educating surgeons may well find the new generation of surgeons arriving with personal values which differ from their own, and being influenced by new institutional values endemic to a rapidly changing NHS. It is essential that those who have been in practice for some time create an understanding between themselves and the younger members of the profession on how these changes will affect all their clinical lives. Without establishing such an agreed understanding, the expectations of both teachers and learners in surgical practice may be seriously unfulfilled.

Further explorations of professional values

This section offers four approaches to considering the significance of values and how they underpin professional practice. Any or all of these could be used as resources by surgeon educators to help them to think more deeply about their own values, and to encourage young surgeons to do the same. This section begins with a model which emphasizes two very different ways of seeing the world of professional practice. Secondly, it explores what it means to be a member of a profession and the values to which those who belong to a profession inevitably subscribe. Thirdly, it offers one way of setting out professional values in surgery, and finally, it provides an extract from the RCS Eng's Curriculum Framework for SHO education in which the College lists the professional values it wishes to see inform the education of surgeons (RCS Eng, 2003).

Two models of professional practice and their values

Readers should be aware, as they consider the following, that models are dangerous because they are reductionist, and that their chief use is in stimulating discussion. The following polemical models present two pictures of professional practice in order to explore their views and the values that underpin them. Readers should critique the following, and consider their own position in respect of it. Is there a middle way which is cohesive in its arguments and characterized by as clear a logic as the following? Or must the espousal of some elements of one lead to a rejection of the other? (Our view is that technical skills are necessary but not sufficient as the basis for professional practice.)

Professional practice is conceived of by some people as involving a set of clear-cut routines and behaviours (performances) and a pre-packaged content which requires merely an efficient means of delivery. They argue (value the idea) that this cuts down considerably on the risk that professionals might fail to provide a reliable service. In turn, this makes assumptions that practice is a relatively simple interaction in which the practitioner knows what should happen, despite appearing to negotiate with patients or clients. However, this view is seen by others as denying the real character of both professionalism on the one hand and practice on the other. Such people value, and therefore argue for the importance of, complex decision-making and elements of professional judgement and practical wisdom guided by moral principles. These they see as central to the daily work of professional practitioners, which cannot be set down in absolute routines.

The first view of professionalism is known as the Technical Rational (TR) view (see Schön, 1987). It characterizes professional activities as essentially simple, describable and able to be broken down into their component parts (skills) and finally mastered. It sees a professional as being essentially efficient in skills which they harness in order to carry out other people's decisions. Another term for 'skills' is 'competencies'. In this view, practitioners are accountable for a set of competencies within their defined area of practice. However, this means that they are answerable only for the technical accuracy of their work, within the bounds of achieving other people's goals. Thus, in the TR view, the professional's role becomes purely instrumental, and some would argue that this reduces the work of a professional to a sub-professional level.

The second view, the Professional Artistry (PA) view (see Schön, 1987), defines behaving professionally as being concerned with both means and ends. (It is concerned with conduct rather than mere behaviour.) Here, professional activity is more akin to artistry, and practitioners are broadly autonomous, making their own decisions, and, essentially, exercising their professional judgement both about their actions and the moral bases of those actions. In this model the professional is not less accountable. Here, to be professional is to be morally accountable for all one's conduct (not just the delivery of the service). Conduct, then, rather than performance, becomes of central value.

In the PA view, professional judgement is neither a simple skill, nor is it able to be subdivided into a series of simple skills. In fact, this view of professional practice, whilst seeing professional skills as necessary, recognizes that they alone are not a sufficient descriptor of professional practice. In fact, it argues, professional activity includes components which cannot be entirely disentangled and treated separately. The PA view of practice, then, takes (and values) a more holistic view. It is concerned with competence. (We discuss the distinction between competence and competencies in detail in Chapter 6.)

Each view of professional expertise brings with it a different view of (set of values about) what professionals should do in order to learn and then to continue to develop their practice.

Those who subscribe to a TR view argue that professional practice has now advanced to the point where goals can be set by society for professionals whose role is purely instrumental. Examples of this can be seen in the very language of health care today, including 'clinical guidelines; clinical outcomes; health outcome individualization; health technology assessment; all of which form part of NHS strategies for improving the effectiveness of the service it provides' (Culshaw, 1995, p.233). The view here is that the professional's role can now be entirely analyzed in terms of activities and skills, and that all that remains is to teach these to the professional trainee. From this set of values, then, it is possible to argue that to learn professional practice is to identify and then to practise skills until they have been mastered, and then to learn to apply them with success to real situations. The language here is about competencies (each skill being a competency). In this view, to improve practice is to move on to harder skills and more complex situations (this is an incremental view of practice). The fact that many of these competencies are simple and can be quickly taught, simply practised and easily measured or observed is also regarded as entirely desirable in a world of diminishing resources.

By contrast, however, those subscribing to the PA view would argue that describing practice in terms of simple pre-set routines and procedures, skills and knowledge, does not do justice to the real experience of professional practice. They value and would emphasize the messy, unpredictable, and unexpected nature of practice, where the ability to improvise is vital. (It is an irony, for example, that an ability to improvise is often diminished by training and routine, yet all practice that is not conveyer-belt repetition involves some improvisation.) This view also values the ability of the practitioner autonomously to be able to refine and update his/her expertise 'on the hoof', rather than needing 're-training'.

The problem seen with the TR approach to professional practice is that it leads to an obsessive intention to tie things down further and further in the inevitably vain attempt to try to cater for all eventualities. By contrast, the PA view values a professional who has been educated roundly, not drilled in skills. In this view, to improve practice is to treat it more holistically, to work to understand its complexities (as well as refining the skills it requires). It seeks a practitioner who knows how and when to use those skills. It values looking carefully at one's actions and theories as one works, and challenging them with ideas from other perspectives, and seeking to improve and refine both practice and its underlying theory. In the PA view, then, the professional is working towards increased competence. Such competence is of course grounded in skills, but not to the exclusion of wider capabilities.

Thus, the TR view values the centrality of rules, schedules, prescriptions, whereas the PA view values the idea that practice starts where the rules fade (because the rules rarely fit real practice). The PA view relies on frameworks and rules of thumb, rather than rules. The TR view emphasizes diagnosis, analysis, and efficient systems. It values the idea of being able to analyze a professional role down to the last detail. The PA view by contrast, believes instead in interpretation of these details, and acknowledges the inevitable subjectivity of setting them down. It comes to an understanding of professional activities by means of appreciation (recognizing the elements which conduce to the overall unity and impact, as in the critical appreciation of art and music). It values and wishes to encourage not narrow efficiency but professional creativity and the right to be wrong. While the TR model assumes that knowledge is permanent, able to be totally mastered, and thus worth attempting to master, the PA view is that knowledge is temporary, dynamic and problematic, and that knowing processes and understanding principles is more useful than knowing facts and learning skills alone.

The TR view values only 'formal theory' produced by researchers (who stand apart from the practitioners). Such formal theory is to be learnt and then applied to practice. Practice is regarded as the arena in which to demonstrate previously worked-out theory. However, this makes for problems when practice becomes more complex and human in its demands.

By contrast, the PA view values also the theory that is implicit in (underlies) all action, and argues that both action and theory are developed in practice, that refining practice involves unearthing the theories on which it is founded and that formal theory aids the development of practice by challenging and extending the practitioner's understandings. The PA view is that (with the help of reflection), theory also emerges *from* practice.

Table 2:2 The technical rational and professional artistry views of professionalism (see Fish and Twin, 1997, p. 45).

The technical rational view	The professional artistry view
Follows rules, laws, routines and prescriptions	Starts where rules fade, and sees patterns, uses frameworks
Uses diagnosis and analysis	Also uses interpretation and appreciation
Seeks efficient systems	Seeks creativity and room to be wrong
Sees knowledge as graspable, permanent	Knowledge is seen as temporary, dynamic, and problematic
Theory is applied to practice	Theory also emerges from practice
Visible performance is central	There is more to professional practice than the surface features
Setting out, and testing for, competency is vital	There is more to professional practice than the sum of its parts
Technical expertise is all	Professional judgement counts
Sees professional activities as 'masterable'	Sees mystery at the heart of professional activities
Emphasizes the known	Embraces uncertainty
Standards must be fixed, standards are measurable, and must be controlled	That which is most easily fixed and measurable is also often trivial. Professionals should be trusted
Emphasizes assessment, appraisal, inspection, accreditation	Emphasizes investigation, reflection, deliberation
Change must be managed from outside	Professionals can develop from inside
Quality is really about the quantity of that which is easily measurable	Quality comes from deepening insight into one's own values, priorities, actions
This is about technical accountability	This is about professional answerability
This requires training	This requires education
This takes the instrumental view	This sees professional work as intrinsically worthwhile

The TR view argues for the mastery of skills and uses the erroneous claim that skills are 'generic' (implying that they transfer), in order to justify teaching them as if they can be unproblematically utilized in all contexts. By contrast, the PA view holds to the notion that skills will always need to be adapted to each new context, even if the routinized craft skills on which artistry is based are able to be specified, and that only principles are truly generic, being flexible tenets, not rigid rules. The PA view of human activity, is that there is always some mystery at its heart, and that the conduct of the professional is not entirely able to be analyzed down to the last atom. It values the notion that professional practitioners are eternal seekers rather than 'knowers'. And it sees the activities of the professional as mainly open capacities which cannot be mastered, which involve creativity on the spot, and which thus inevitably involve risk (there being no creativity without risk). It also recognizes that learning to do is only achieved by engaging in action, together with reflecting upon the action, and where improvisation, enquiry into action and resulting insight by those involved in it, generate a major knowledge base.

Each model also gives rise to a particular view of, and way of valuing quality. The TR model uses the language of quality control. It places emphasis upon visible performance and seeks to test and measure these, valuing technical expertise as all-important and the idea that learning results in immediately visible products. Thus, the model is behaviourist, and emphasizes fixed standards, and ways of controlling these.

By contrast, the PA view values more than the surface and visible features of professional practice. It believes that there is more to the whole than the sum of the parts, it values the central role of professional judgement, and holds that the most easily measurable is often also the most trivial. Further, it values investigation, reflection and deliberation as a means to enable professionals to develop their own insights from inside, and holds that this is a better means of staff development than innovation imposed from outside. In short, it sees quality as coming from deepening insight into one's own values, priorities and actions.

Table 2:2 offers a summary of the points above.

Membership of a profession

The word 'profession' is still the only precise term for characterizing specialist groups who earn a particular kind of living in an exchange economy. Being a member of a profession is far more than merely behaving professionally (which is often used to imply that people are efficient, punctual or well presented). Far beyond this, membership of a profession commits an individual to subscribe to those general values that are found across all professions.

Members of a profession work in practical human settings in which they offer a valuable 'good', or well-being, to individuals and society, which is of such value that money cannot serve as its sole measure. Their preparation for their livelihood, their motivation to join their profession, and their continuing professional development, separate them from other groups who earn a living. Thus, even in the 21st Century, their work is different in kind as well as in degree from that of other occupations.

Being a member of a profession therefore involves engaging in an occupation, which may be characterized as follows.

- ❏ It is complex, and so, in the public interest, practitioners need to be educated and assessed by members of their profession in order to enter that profession. To continue within it, they must now be prepared to engage in life-long development.
- ❏ Professional practitioners identify closely with their work, such that they develop intellectual interests in it.
- ❏ The work of a member of a profession takes place in practical settings, which require the use of esoteric, theoretical knowledge; a researched base; and high level skill (none of which a lay-person can entirely obtain, totally comprehend or fully evaluate).
- ❏ It involves working with people who are vulnerable, and thus demands the professional practitioner's acknowledgement of moral and ethical considerations.
- ❏ The human situations in which professionals work involve some unpredictability, and so not every element of the work of a professional can be predetermined.
- ❏ Because every person for whom professionals work is particular and individual, professionals must use their judgement. Thus, the work of a professional is discretionary in nature.
- ❏ This in turn requires that practitioners have self-knowledge and are aware of their own personal and professional values and the values of their profession.
- ❏ 'Confidentiality', 'etiquette' and 'collegiality' are important concepts in the work of a professional practitioner.
- ❏ Their work requires practitioners to operate within the bounds and traditions of the profession through which they are licensed to practice. Such traditions have been developed over a long period in response to the demands and values of society.
- ❏ Professional bodies are the guardians of these standards, and as such are regulatory.

Professionals 'accept being members of a professional society where questions, dilemmas and the implications of new findings are continuously discussed' (Stiwne and Abrandt Dahlgren, 2004, p. 160).

Current demands upon professionals to achieve performance targets are leading to the erosion of these traditional ways of working and being. We would argue that the demotivation of senior members of professions, many of whom are set to leave their practice prematurely, is probably related to this. Young professionals, those considering such a career, and those involved in their education, need to give careful thought to this changing world and its effect on the development of the professional practitioner of the future.

Many professions have already recognized that they will fail the public if they allow these crucial characteristics to be obscured and undervalued. Where this is the case, they have built consideration of such matters into their curriculum at all levels. Where it is not the case, the profession is in danger of losing its character, its ability to provide a high level service for the public and ultimately, its standing in society.

Two examples of professional values

The following two examples (example one, Figure 2:3; and example two) demonstrate the articulation of professional values which have been developed by surgeons. The first was an early attempt to find a way of presenting the three main areas in which professional values are most influential, and to make it clear that patients were at the centre of this. The second, comes from the draft 'Curriculum for the General Professional Practice of Surgery' for SHO education (piloted by the Royal College of Surgeons of England in 2003). It will be clear from the following that in development from Figure 2:3 to the second example, a non-diagrammatic form was adopted, and the three headings were reduced to two and presented in a text format only.

Example one: a version of professional values

Strong personal organisation

A commitment to operative excellence

An ability to exercise sound professional judgement

The ability to lead

The ability to think 'on their feet' and the ability to think, do and talk at the same time

An ability to continuously develop their practice through reflection

An ability to share knowledge and ability with others in surgery

An ability to operate with some autonomy within the acceptable limits of the profession

A recognition that the patient should be considered holistically

A commitment to lifelong learning

A commitment to a professional life of accountability

PROFESSIONAL PRACTICE   **PROFESSIONAL DEVELOPMENT**   **PATIENT CARE**

A sensitivity to moral and ethical issues implicit in their practice which are current in society

A commitment to patient-centred practice

An ability to inform, educate and manage patient expectations

An ability to engage in the development of the profession

A criticality towards skills, knowledge and know-how

An ability to exercise practical wisdom through reflection and deliberation

An ability to recognize the incompleteness and temporary nature of professional work and to be able to live and work in this environment

An ability to work in collaboration with colleagues and patients

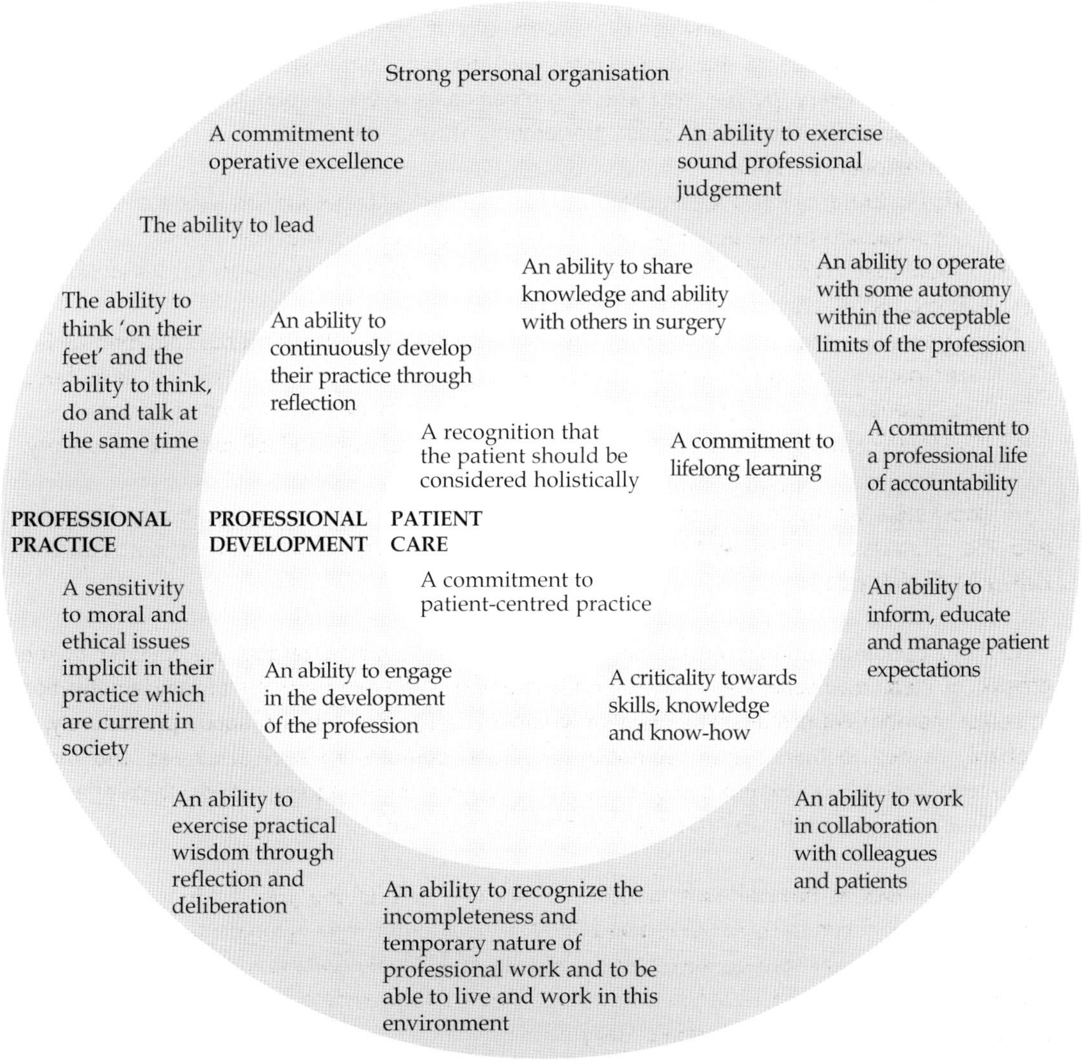

Figure 2:3 An early version of the RCS Eng's professional values (RCS Eng, 2001). (Reprinted with permission from The Royal College of Surgeons of England.)

Example two: an extract from the Royal College of Surgeons of England's Draft Curriculum Framework for SHO education (RCS Eng, 2003, pp. 3-4)

Professional obligations to patients involve:

- a commitment to a partnership of care;
- recognition of the whole person within their social, ethical and cultural context;
- the honouring of the relationship of trust with the patient with its concomitant moral and ethical responsibilities; and
- a dedication to clear, honest and empathetic communication.

Professional practice and professional development involves:

- A commitment to:
  - ❖ clinical and operative excellence;
  - ❖ a professional life and the responsibilities that this implies, especially those of accountability;
  - ❖ lifelong learning and professional self-development; and
  - ❖ continuous questioning, deliberation and reflection in developing new professional knowledge and understanding.

- Recognition that:
  - ❖ surgeons perform operations on patients as a necessary part of their care and in that respect differ from many other doctors;
  - ❖ the dynamic nature of professional knowledge, and the ability to work in this environment requires the recognition of personal limits; and
  - ❖ the practice of surgery draws upon both the knowledge and use of science as well as sound professional artistry.

- The ability to:
  - ❖ work with a degree of autonomy but within the parameters set and monitored by the profession;
  - ❖ engage in the development of the profession as a whole by sharing knowledge and understanding to influence and change practice;
  - ❖ respect and work in collaboration with colleagues;
  - ❖ lead where appropriate; and
  - ❖ focus on the salient features of practice and exercise wisdom.

- Sensitivity to the moral and ethical issues implicit in surgical practice in contemporary society.

These values conform to the spirit of both *Good Medical Practice* (GMC, 2001), and *Good Surgical Practice* (RCS Eng, 2002).

The use and significance of professional values in teaching and learning in clinical settings

Teachers are models of professional values, in the sense that their activities and the values which lie under them are visible to all with whom they engage in educational and clinical matters. They cannot but offer themselves as an example of 'how to be' in clinical settings.

What it means for the teacher as professional

This means that their conduct is inevitably under constant scrutiny and is open to interpretation by all who observe it. For example, in any clinical situation, the patient, the nurse, the secretary, the learner, and other surgical colleagues, as part of the wider community of practice, will observe the teacher from differing perspectives. They will naturally compare and contrast the teacher's values with their own and with the various values statements of the wider health care communities of which they are all a part.

Surgical teachers working in complex clinical environments lead both clinical and educational processes. They are responsible for overseeing the harmonising of complex situations involving many groups, each with different requirements. The smooth running of such a process might seem effortless and easy to an uninformed observer. There is a danger that the learning surgeon may try to *copy* rather than *understand* how this was achieved.

This places on the teacher the responsibility of ensuring that the learning surgeon understands the processes and motivations that have allowed this activity to appear effortless. The teacher must therefore value the opportunity to deliberate with the learner about how they have achieved this and encourage the learner to understand how they might fine-tune their own response to the conflicting demands that they will meet in their own clinical practice.

What it means for the learner

Learners too are models of professional values, and their conduct, like that of their teacher, is under constant scrutiny from many perspectives. They are at the same time both learners and surgical practitioners. Those observing their conduct will inevitably make comparisons between themselves and the learner. The potential for unpacking the values of the learner offers both educator and learner a more profound opportunity for educational development than is currently recognized.

The learner has to recognize that values as well as knowledge underpin the actions of the teacher and the surgeon. This will involve the learner in both understanding their own motivations (what drives their learning and their practice), and those of their teacher/surgeon. Development of the learner is not about copying but about understanding and this is something to be valued by both the teacher and the learner.

Chapter 3

The importance in postgraduate medicine of educational values, principles and aims

Introduction

The current context of postgraduate medical education and the basis for our critique

Postgraduate medical education currently

What is education, and what is an educational practice?

Knowledge organization and generation: a matter of power and its use

Educational values and their importance for teachers and learners

The contrasting values endemic to education and training

The educational values and principles that surgeons might embrace

The significant decisions teachers make

End note

Introduction

The intentions of this chapter, like those of the book as a whole, are challenging - even radical. We seek to offer surgeons an *informed* choice about how to work with postgraduate doctors to enable them to become surgeons. We seek to contribute a voice which will engender educational thought and debate. This will involve a comment on current postgraduate medical education, a consideration of different ways of thinking about how to support postgraduate doctors as they learn their practice, and a contribution to new ways forward.

The current context of postgraduate medical education and the basis for our critique

This section uses comments on current postgraduate medical education as a springboard for providing, in two subsections, critical scrutiny of the key educational thinking that underlies those comments. It thus seeks to offer readers emancipation from the present thinking, which we believe has emanated from political rather more than educational concerns. It will therefore undoubtedly challenge surgeons' current ways of thinking about, and engaging in, education in clinical settings.

Postgraduate medical education currently

We welcome the moves in *Modernising Medical Careers* (MMC) (Department of Health and Social Security, 2002, 2003 and 2004), towards enabling postgraduate doctors to learn and be assessed more rigorously *in the clinical setting*. We endorse the idea that every demand of service provides an educational opportunity from which new doctors need to learn (and to know how to learn). We share the notion that new doctors need to be part of service rather than supernumerary. We recognize the educational obligations of all doctors (GMC, 1999). We believe that a national level initiative was necessary. What needs to support all this (and is currently lacking however), is:

- ❏ an *educationally* sound curriculum framework; and
- ❏ strong support for teachers and learners to adopt educational understanding of, and therefore appropriate new approaches to, teaching and assessing in clinical settings.

Although it is aimed primarily at surgeons, this book offers help in discussing the detail of educating all doctors in clinical thinking, clinical knowledge and clinical processes. Fish and Coles (forthcoming) offers new ways forward in developing a curriculum for medical practice.

Already, in the pilots of Foundation Year Two (F2), the green shoots of educational *possibility* are appearing. But without proper educational support as indicated above, we believe, this important initiative will gain only patchy hold, and will rapidly regress to older, less appropriate activities which will not make the best capital out of the investment in it of energy, time and other resources. Neither will it provide quality education, better prepared doctors, nor a good basis for the further postgraduate development of the medical profession.

The practices being advocated, or rather required, in the F2 curriculum currently, are mainly drawn from training not education (and are thus concerned with surface performance rather than morally informed conduct). The political reasons for this include the idea that training will achieve many short-term goals fast. No one explains that the ultimate cost will be greater in the longer term, as changes in performance are neither properly implemented nor do they provide for future development. Those in control claim that there is no time or resource to engage in education. But we would argue that it is the other way round. We (and many like us) believe that medicine in Britain in the 21st Century cannot afford *not* to find the time and resource for education.

Accordingly, this chapter seeks to provide the educational understanding out of which surgical teachers can develop, articulate and defend their own coherent, logical and cohesive educational practice, and thus regain the initiative of developing their profession. It does so by illustrating and exploring a range of alternative values which have specific relevance to surgical education and the fact that it takes place in clinical settings.

The main thinking which underlies the rest of this chapter offers a radically different way of seeing, understanding and engaging in developing postgraduate doctors. It is as follows.

What is education, and what is an educational practice?

There is a logic that is central to educational thinking, without consideration of which no activity can legitimately claim to be educational. This logic can be illustrated as follows.

1. **Education is an ethical activity**, undertaken in pursuit of educationally worthwhile ends and which seeks to realize morally worthwhile virtues. The following offers a range of ways of thinking about this.

    For example, educational practice is 'morally informed and morally committed action' (see Carr, 1995, pp. 64 and 68). The role of the educator is to facilitate the process of growth in the learner (to enhance individual freedom, develop autonomy and contribute to democracy (see the work of Dewey). Education liberates individuals and facilitates their transition from passive to active learners. It is emancipatory, cannot be morally neutral, is always directive (but the ends and means used can be liberating), is a social process and above all is the practice of freedom in which learners discover themselves and achieve their humanity (see the work of Freire). (By now it will be clear that being a professional practice, education has important theoretical underpinnings.)

    An important dimension here relates to the relationship between power and knowledge, which we will explore in the following section.

2. These **worthwhile ends, aims or goals** of education include the development of the whole person and particularly the cultivation of the mind (which means developing understanding which in turn will lead to the development of practice). That is, educators seek to extend the learner's *understanding*, because where understanding is developed in learners, they will then choose to change their conduct accordingly and will be responsible for, and genuinely committed to, that change, and have the motivation and capability to continue to develop it. This constitutes a major educational aim. Logically, (if the enterprise is to be counted as education) consideration of such aims must come before all other decisions about how to teach, learn, assess, and evaluate. The expression of these aims is always shaped by underlying values which need to be transparent and which the educator is inevitably promoting through that expression.

3. The puzzle for the educator, then, is how best to develop in learners this kind of understanding. For example, two key processes in this are: to engage them in critical thinking and to support them in making their own meaning from their experiences. (These are means to achieve that aim, end or goal.) To ask what learners and teachers generally need to do to engage learners in this, is to ask: what **principles of procedure** should guide their activities? However, to argue for the significance of educational principles is not the same as wanting to turn them into a set of codified rules to be followed slavishly. In fact, the value of educational principles is that they guide practice in general terms but do not shape and control it in the specific case.

4.   To choose **particular activities**, of teaching, learning and assessment, which are tailored to the individual learner's needs as construed and agreed by both teacher and learner, is to make wise judgements which will then lead to **sound educational action**.

Note: the *logic* here is precisely the same as that of the diagnostic process that doctors engage in. They formulate the patient's clinical problem, explore this and come to a general clinical solution, which they then have to tailor to the individual patient's case in order to come to an agreed treatment plan. That is, the *principles* of clinical thinking and those of educational thinking are the same. Readers who wish to explore this in more detail are invited to consider the elements of clinical thinking we offer (on page 137), and how these cash out into a diagnostic pathway (page 155 and Figure 7.3 on page 158).

5.   **A practice cannot be claimed as educational unless it is underpinned by (implicit or explicit) understanding of what it is 'to act educationally'.** It is broadly agreed by educators that to act educationally is to open minds, liberate thinking, encourage critique, explore the foundations of good practice and develop creativity (see as key authors the work of Peters, Oakeshott, Carr, W., Dewey, Freire, Rogers, Habermas, Van Manen, Faucault).

Where the activity engaged in does open minds, liberate thinking, encourage critique and so on, practitioners may, irrespective of their know-how or skills, claim to practise in an educational way (see Carr, 1995, p. 160). Where it is not so, no amount of teaching skills will compensate, and no technical know-how will make the experience educational for learners.

6.   **Education is 'a practice'** because these ends and virtues can only be realized through, and exist in, action, and they are themselves being continuously developed. That is, learners are not artifacts that can be made, or turned into the ideal end-product. You cannot make a thinking surgeon, you can only seek to cultivate one. And in so doing, you cannot precisely specify the ends of such cultivation. One cannot specify in April, the precise character of the roses that will spring in July from the bush one is then pruning. One can work towards shaping the bush, and one can hope for given colour and growth, but one cannot say more.

7.   Why then are we endlessly badgered to specify 'learning outcomes' that nail down every last detail of what the learner will be able to do at the end of the programme even before it begins, and that often lead to predictability and boredom for learner and reduce the teacher's room for creativity? It is because this way of thinking springs from **a quite different view of preparing practitioners**, which is based upon the values of training rather than education, and which rejects the notion that the 'growth metaphor' is a suitable analogy for an activity which is seen as mainly about being drilled in skills, so as to be safe practitioners. But, in fact, such drilling (which saves practitioners from thinking) may result in more danger to patients in complex individual cases where careful thought and complex decisions are needed, and where doctors actually need to use their judgement.

8. As Carr shows, **to engage in an educational practice is more than about 'knowing how to do educational things'** (having the skills of teaching). Indeed, an educational method (like instructing doctors in a given skill) can be skillfully performed but it will not be an educational practice at all, if (for example), it has been used to impose a process upon learners who have been required to ignore their personal perspectives including their own values, attitudes and feelings, suspend their thinking, shut down their critical faculties, abandon their moral awareness, and merely parrot a performance. This would not conform to ethical educational principles of procedure concerned with cultivating the understanding which enables learners to explore and come to own a view about why, how, where and when to use that skill, which in turn commits them to develop or change their practice. Indeed, it would be training (which we explore below).

9. Of course, it is clear that **in surgery, craft skills will have to be learnt** and this will require some elements of training. Beyond this, however, surgical teaching could be shaped either by the notion of training or education. Those who see surgeons as mainly technical experts will value and wish to argue for skills-based training which is largely concerned with learning new behaviour (procedures and operations). Those who seek to cultivate a surgeon who is aware of the importance of professional judgement and who knows when, where and how to utilize those skills in the health care setting and who does so with sensitivity and humanity, will argue for education which is concerned with changing (deepening) understanding as a basis for intelligent skills and well considered conduct. It will be clear from this that we do not regard training in skills as sufficient to support the development of a thinking surgeon.

So far we have said little about knowledge. As indicated above, there is a further dimension to these arguments, which concerns the relationship between knowledge and power.

Knowledge organization and generation: a matter of power and its use

It will be clear from the above argument there are still choices to be made by teachers in their own contexts within the broad educational aims we have outlined. The role of the teacher is very powerful. In making their choices they must decide: whose knowledge is to be taught; how it should be construed; where they believe it is created; and to what end it is to be offered to, or facilitated in, learners. Even in deciding *not* to exercise this choice and accepting that made for them by others, teachers are shaping (or rather short-changing) their own and their learner's educational possibilities.

The work of Habermas helps us to understand this. Drawing on his ideas, Grundy (1987) identified three systems of knowledge generation and organisation: the technical; the practical; and the emancipatory. Habermas's 'technical approach' is concerned with questions about what the practical worker should do on the spot. It seeks to improve outcomes by improving skills. This approach allows knowledge to be controlled by one group within health care and sees success in terms of effectiveness and efficiency. Here, theory directs, confirms and legitimates practice. This is what we have earlier called the technical rational approach. Those who follow it practise according to rules and use their skills to a pre-determined end.

By contrast, Habermas's 'practical approach' sees practice as guided by choice, which in turn is guided by a disposition towards what is 'good'. This involves an aspect of moral consciousness. There is greater choice here for the practitioner. The practitioner would break rules if s/he judged it necessary for good. Here, the practical decisions have to be made in the actual situation. This involves what he calls 'practical judgement' which is exercised through deliberation (or reflection). Further, as well as knowledge arising directly through reflection upon practice, Habermas's 'practical interest' encourages the development of knowledge through the bringing to consciousness of implicit theory, thus providing a more consciously rational basis for action.

The third or 'emancipatory approach' to generating and organising knowledge, engages students in the active creation of knowledge along with the teacher. Here, teaching and learning are regarded as problematic, the teacher is taught in a dialogue along with the student, and theory and practice must both be open to critical scrutiny. Dialogue is a vital means of learning, and a curriculum is not a written plan but an active process in which planning, acting and evaluating are reciprocally related. The word 'critique' is taken to mean a more fundamental questioning of both theory and practice than is found in the practical approach and than is meant in the traditional use of the term 'critical thinking'.

In setting out these categories, Grundy distinguishes between 'reproductive' and radically 'transformative' approaches to education.

She argues that the emancipatory approach provides for authentic learning by students as opposed to the 'co-opted agreement' which characterizes other approaches (Grundy, 1987, p. 125). Here, knowledge is socially constructed, the teacher recognizes 'moral constraint in the extent to which student learning may be coerced' (and the learner can thus control the learning situation). The locus of control for making judgements about the quality and meaningfulness of the work lie with the participants in the learning situation and there is freedom to question accepted wisdom, recognize that things are not as they seem to be and develop a sophisticated critical consciousness where questioning leads to investigation which leads to critical insight. This authentic critique 'looks back at theory and, while trying to make meaning of it, critically examines its value for practice' (Grundy, 1987, p. 132). Here, theory provides information but not direction. This approach brings enlightenment and transforms consciousness, enabling us to see the constraints around our practice and to break out of habitual ways of seeing things and of acting.

Table 3:1 shows this in detail (but it should be remembered that this is a mere summary of complex and closely argued work which can best be pursued by readers through Grundy, 1987; and Fish and Coles, 1998). Although these ideas are presented by Grundy as illuminating education more generally, our summary casts Habermas's argument in terms of education for the professions. In preparation for the next section readers might like to ask themselves what values imbue the following.

Readers might wish to return to this when they reach Chapters 7 and 8.

Table 3:1 A summary of the arguments of Habermas.

The questions	The technical approach	The practical approach	The emancipatory approach
	Teacher inculcates those skills which society needs and government has decided to require of professionals. (How these have been decided may or may not have been democratic)	Teacher is a thinking agent of what those in power require of professionals, but may act partially independently for the good of learners and even the profession	Teacher is an educator who takes informed and critical responsibility for the ends and the means of the education s/he offers and who seeks to enable learners to do the same, both in education and in their own profession
What approach should teacher take?	Enact a curriculum which has been handed down	Choose what will bring about learners' good	Enable learners to create knowledge along with teacher
Teacher's intention	To improve outcomes by improving skills	To develop understanding and moral consciousness	To enable learners to see that teaching and learning are problematic
Who controls the knowledge during learning?	Whoever controls the teacher's ideas about what must be taught (one group only, which is outside the teaching/ learning interaction)	The teacher chooses what is learnt during practice, but can break the rules for the good of the learner and all have equal rights within the situation	Teacher and learner learn together in dialogue. Dialogue is a vital means of learning. Knowledge is a corporate matter, created *in situ*
What is the role of educational theory in this?	Theory (from outside, which is formal, but already chosen by the control group) directs and confirms practice	A range of theory is drawn on by teacher which guides meaning-making in a democratic environment, and enables personal theory, belief, and assumption to be exhumed and examined	Theory (of all kinds) and practice, are questioned fundamentally. A critique is developed while trying to make meaning of both theory and practice
What judgements (decisions) may teachers make in practice?	They may decide only how to attain an end which has been stipulated by someone else who is not part of the teaching situation (strategic judgement)	They may engage personal judgement about the practicalities of teaching (the means to be used) through reflection, deliberation, and critical thinking. They have no choice about ends (practical judgement)	They can use own judgement about ends and means by understanding the choices that may be made and by careful deliberation about them and critique of them (professional judgement)
Teacher's role	Totally reproductive of what has been decided by others	Essentially reproductive of what has been decided by others	Emancipatory. Brings enlightenment and transforms consciousness and self-awareness

Our own values as authors incline us to Habermas's arguments. (These we hold because we have clarified them, but we also seek to challenge, refine and develop them continuously.) In order to equip readers with a more fully informed base from which to shape their own philosophies, the values and practices of both education and training will be considered in the following sections, together with the current traditions of teaching in surgical settings and their educational values, and some new perspectives on these matters.

Educational values and their importance for teachers and learners

We have argued that developing thinking surgeons requires teachers whose educational practice is logical, coherent, morally informed, and can be articulated and eternally revised and re-interpreted. Such practice needs, we argue, to be underpinned by a sound, coherent and logical educational philosophy, beneath which lie transparent and cohesive personal and educational values. These need to result in clear and defensible educational principles.

That is why, in this book, we seek to cultivate surgical teachers who have the understanding and ability to build their own educational philosophy, which is logical and ethical. In order to begin this life-time enterprise, they will need to have considered critically the choices available to them (and the terms in which we present them). They will then need to be able to clarify and defend their own values whilst always keeping an open mind by holding them as temporary. Accordingly, we now offer the detail about the differing values of education and training and why they are important.

The contrasting values endemic to education and training

As authors, we have declared our educational ends, as if this is a straightforward matter with which everyone would agree. But there is no one universally agreed answer to any educational question. Everything about education is problematic because it is values-based and the answers to educational questions are imbued with the values held by those who answer. The aims (ends or goals) of education are thus endlessly contestable.

The way that aims are articulated depends upon the values, and educational understanding of the person formulating them. This is important because those values also shape the ensuing activities of teacher and learner (including the use of reflection on practice - see Chapter 5; and the role of assessment in learning, which we consider in detail in Chapter 6).

For example, to value above all else the visible performance of a surgeon, is to subscribe to the view that learning is about changing or learning new behaviour. Such a view might at first sight be attractive, but only if one wishes to promote a narrow aim, one that can be attended to by training rather than education, and which will focus on the teacher drilling the learner in actions. Here, the teacher's instructional and presentational skills are important, and the learner's ability involves precise copying. The end result of this will be a technician who can apply these skills to practice, but only by replicating them exactly, and who cannot adapt this know-how to new contexts, and does not understand how, why, when and where it is appropriate to deploy them.

By contrast, to value in a practitioner 'conduct which is morally shaped', casts learning as 'a comprehensive activity in which we come to know ourselves and the world around us'. Here, the teaching is valued as opening up to learners their wide inheritance and extending the learner's (and the teacher's own) criticality in every aspect of their work, as well as challenging the very bases for that criticality (ways of seeing the world of practice). (See Oakeshott, 1967, p. 120.) This will lead to educational activities that focus more on what it is *worthwhile* for the learner to do, than on the teacher's skills, more on a collaborative approach to learning, than on teacher as agent of someone else's change, and more on thinking practitioners who can defend their actions and recognize their moral dimensions than on technicians who simply do as they have been taught.

Where many educational philosophers see learning as a change in *understanding*, and education as the development of the mind, behavoural psychologists see learning as activity, which leads to a change in *behaviour*, and a reorganization of the learner's habits, skills, knowledge, tendencies, and his/her relationship with his/her environment. Training thus values skills and measurable behaviour to the exclusion of all else. 'A world that cannot be perceived, explained and measured is deemed [by trainers] to be either unimportant or non-existent' (Broadfoot, 2000, p. 199). Such learning, at base, involves a response to a stimulus. It thus puts the teacher (stimulator) in control, and gives the learner little choice about either what will be learnt or how. The sign of such learning is a change in performance, which is visible and measurable. A pure form of this kind of teaching involves repeated provision by teacher of stimuli calculated to affect the overt activity of the learner, but without the learner engaging in thought about that activity. A famous simple example is Pavlov's dogs who were trained to salivate when a bell was rung because the bell was presented whenever their food appeared until the dogs responded to the bell in the absence of food.

Training engages the learner in physically copying required behaviour, rather than engaging the mind with any moral concerns related to how such behaviour might be used, or with any critical perspectives on the teaching and learning involved. The person who requires and values that new behaviour is the teacher (not necessarily the learner). Learners, in this view, have little control over their own destiny and teaching verges on indoctrination whose definition, arguably, refers to the gross manipulation of the learner.

For trainers who follow behavioural psychology, satisfactory learning is signified by new behaviour. See, for example: 'Change is what learning is all about, and a widely accepted view would equate learning with a change in the behaviour of an organism which persists over time' (Stones, 1979, p. 7). The derivation of many of these ideas can be traced through early psychologists like Skinner, through the work of Tyler, (1949), which is significantly focused on the basic principles of curriculum and instruction, and culminates in the work of Bloom, (1956), a handbook, which contains the famous Taxonomy of Educational Objectives for the cognitive domain, and Krathwohl *et al*, (1964), which provides the handbook which classifies all the learning goals for the affective domain.

The work of Stones in teacher education (which has not met with universal popularity, but has probably shaped the competency-based approach to today's Department for Education and Science requirements on teachers in training), illustrates how these ideas can emerge in practice. He produced three protocols (though he did not use this term). These were: Schedule for the Teaching of Psycho-motor Skills (STOPS); Schedule for the Teaching and Evaluation of Problem Solving (STEPS), and a Schedule for Evaluating Teaching (SET).

In the first of these (STOPS), he sets out 'the key aspects of teaching activity to ensure satisfactory learning of psychomotor skills [which] provides a checklist for student teacher and supervisor to evaluate this aspect of teaching'. The protocol consists of three sections. The first is the pre-active stage, where the teacher is required to make a task analysis of the teaching objectives, identify the subordinate skills, decide on methods of presentation, pupils' activities, feedback, and evaluation. The second is the interactive stage, where the task is explained and demonstrated by teacher; the subordinate skills are identified for the learner; the learner describes the activity and guides teacher's performance; the teacher then prompts and guides the learner in carrying out the activities, looking for smooth transition from one sub-skill to the next; the prompts are then faded and the learner gradually assumes responsibility. There is feedback at all stages. The learner practises, and is monitored; and the monitoring is gradually faded. Evaluation is by means of assessing the learner's performance, and the learner's self-assessment (see Stones, 1979, pp. 242-3). A very similar schedule is offered for problem solving. Stones then discusses programmed learning and its Skinnerian basis. (Skinner's work was all on animals, and based on careful programming of the provision of a stimulus, the appearance of a response and the reinforcement of feedback, so as to produce patterns of activity pre-planned by the programmer.)

Readers will doubtless recognize this work as the basis for Training the Trainers. Indeed, it offers one approach to learning skills (though without any attention to when, how and where to use them). What is significant is that Stones shows us how it can be used also for (rather formulaic) problem solving. But he does not attempt to suggest other uses for it. For example, it would be hard to see how it could seriously be used to teach the appreciation of poetry, or indeed any other art. The greatest danger of training then, is to extend it beyond the narrow limits in which it makes sense, or, worse, to dismiss as worthless anything to which it cannot be applied. As Handy says of it quoting MacNamara's fallacy:

'The first step is to measure whatever can easily be measured. This is OK as far as it goes. The second step is to disregard that which can't easily be measured or to give it an arbitrary quantitative value. This is artificial and misleading. The third step is to presume that what can't be measured easily really isn't important. This is blindness. The fourth step is to say that what can't easily be measured really doesn't exist. This is suicide.'

(Handy, 1994, cited by Broadfoot, 2000, p. 219.)

It is true, of course, that training makes quick (cosmetic) changes to practice (which do not last), while education sometimes takes time to show results because new understandings will only gradually influence practitioners' practice, and because new understanding does not necessarily result in immediately adjusted behaviour.

These differences between training and education arise from different ways of seeing what the teacher should engage the learner in, and how and why. As argued in Chapter 2, it seems appropriate to select a teaching approach which best responds to both the character of the professional practice to be learnt and to the nature of the knowledge which the practitioner needs to acquire and draw upon.

To be a member of a health care profession is to possess the necessary knowledge and skills to treat patients, but also to be concerned with moral and ethical matters, and to seek their well-being. It involves making professional judgements on the spot, in practice, rather than simply carrying out some pre-ordained activity without thinking about the particular instance involved. Making such judgements by reading the situation in a particular instance, making meaning out of it and creating at the time a particular response to it based upon theoretical knowledge and the needs of the individual situation, is *not* usually regarded as something one can be trained to do.

Training involves ensuring that the same reaction is always given to a similar event. Soldiers train. Children are trained in certain matters. This is because, for their safety, they must establish unconscious rituals or unthinkingly obey orders instantly. What is valued here is a reliably regular reaction to similar events such that it has become automatic. It may be true that professionals must be trained in the skills and procedures of their craft so that they can reliably reproduce the same standard of skill for all patients, but this is not the same as saying all patients must be treated as if they were exactly the same. Further, a very small amount of professional practice involves trained rituals alone (and even these have been shown to be dangerous to patients if uncritically applied in all cases).

Professionals respond to the patient or event, not by automatically reproducing previous behaviour, but by adapting what they know to the new circumstances of the occasion; that is, society needs professionals to work not routinely, but mindfully. It needs them to act intelligently. This means that they must constantly think about, challenge, and critique what they do. Thus, most of the activities that a member of a profession carries out, need to be underpinned by education not training. Thus, those who foster learning in clinical settings need to extend the learner's and their own criticality, and challenge what they routinely take for granted, seeing their practice in new ways. This will engage the teacher and learner in considering sceptically their most cherished ideas, looking at the moral basis of their decisions and recognizing the costs and benefits and their conflicting values. This is the argument for educating professionals, because education is about deepening understanding (which then affects practice also). It requires teachers who are already insightful and who demonstrate their own drawing together of critical perspectives and even their own uncertainties, as they teach. Such teachers facilitate learning and understanding, and ensure that this is underpinned by activities that enable learners to make their own sense of what they know and do, as they work. To train them would be to ensure that no such critical perspectives and no such moral dimensions exist within their practice.

Thus, we can see that the very language in which we discuss the activities of our teaching and our professional health care practice, carries messages to all interested parties about what we think we are about. (For example, teaching by instructing is very different from facilitating learning.)

The educational values and principles that surgeons might embrace

Clearly, surgeons seek to provide sound educational practice within theatre, ward and clinic. This will take account of the service context, the nature of professional practice, the tacit knowledge and understanding of the consultant surgeon, and the postgraduate educational setting in which doctors learn.

The following educational principles and their associated values are implicit in what we have been saying about an educational practice in clinical settings. Lest what follows should seem overwhelming, we now remind readers of what we said in the introduction, namely that learning the practice of education does not spring fully fledged in the capacities of teachers. It does not need to. A practice is learnt by engaging in it thoughtfully and critically and is illuminated by the ideas of others who are part of the same tradition. Teachers don't need to have developed all these capabilities and perfected them before working with learners. The teaching process is professional development for *both* learner and teacher (that is, unless the teacher aspires to be a trainer in whom all authority rests and whose performance must be a perfect pattern for the trainee!).

It should be noted that, being principles, the following statements are (as we see it) generic to all good educational practice in all surgical contexts. By comparison, skills are not and cannot be generic, being context-specific, and needing to be adapted to each new situation. These principles are offered to stimulate teachers and learners to formulate their own. (They specifically exclude detailed reference to assessment, which we consider in detail in Chapter 6.) As teachers concerned with surgical education we seek to base our work on the following.

- ❐ The practice of education is a moral enterprise, not a technical one.
- ❐ For the practice of teaching to be educational, the aims must be demonstrably worthwhile at the level of developing the whole person.
- ❐ For their practice to be educational, teachers must have considered a range of approaches to teaching, learning and assessment and have made an informed and logical selection from them to suit their aims.
- ❐ The cultivation in the learner of moral awareness is central to education for the professions.
- ❐ The conduct of and justification for education rests on the development of defensible educational values, there being no agreed universal answers and no 'cook-book' guides on how to teach that can guarantee an educational experience for the learner.
- ❐ Surgical teachers as well as learners need to examine their own professional and personal values in order to respond to the competing demands and ethical dilemmas of practice (both educational and health care).
- ❐ All service events are potential learning opportunities.

- The establishment of a learning partnership between teacher and learner is a vital basis for educational practice.
- Respect for the learner, the learner's agenda and the learner's needs to make learning their own, is important.
- Conversation (dialogue) in teaching and learning in surgery is important in that it enables learners to make educational meaning for themselves out of their experiences and their teachers' offerings, and enables teachers to ensure the appropriateness of that 'meaning-making'.
- Establishing an environment that is safe for the patient and nurturing of the learner (within which the learner can then be challenged educationally), is vital to education.
- Facilitating the development of the learner's understanding is a key role for the educator.
- Surgical skills need time for development but they cannot fully be developed outside the clinical setting, and though necessary, they do not, alone, provide a sufficient armamentarium for safe surgical practice.
- Professional judgment is central to both surgery and education, and its development in the learner needs to be attended to specifically.
- Reflection and deliberation provide important means of developing both educational understanding and clinical thinking.
- Criticality is a key characteristic of postgraduate education.
- Self-directed learning and self-assessment are important as ultimate goals for autonomy and liberation from the teacher.
- Learning to work with and communicate with a range of different people is important to all professional education.
- Professionals engage in lifelong learning, and continuous professional development.

The significant decisions teachers make

Trainers offer trainees someone else's agenda, and do so in ways dictated by that agenda, thus having few decisions of their own to make. A teacher, by contrast, engages with a learner in deliberate and planned educational activities about whose ends and means s/he has the power and responsibility to decide. In that sense the current urging to attend only to the development of skills in doctors and surgeons, fits the trend in which we see politicians seeking wherever possible to remove the need for decisions. The pattern is ubiquitous. Politicians currently seek: to determine as many domestic matters as possible on behalf of the man in the street; to save health care professionals as far as possible from making their own decisions by setting up huge machinery for risk-control; to spare school teachers from having to think about what they do with and for pupils, by pre-shaping virtually everything they may do in classrooms; and to reduce to a minimum all professional judgements everywhere, by pressing a skills-based (competency-based) approach to the preparation and development of professionals of all kinds. The bureaucratic mind, of course, is set to follow rule-books and thus to avoid any individual decision-making, which is seen as dangerous, particularly in our present over-litigious society (see also O'Neill, 2002).

By contrast, we believe that on the contrary, not to equip professionals by good education to make sound individual judgements, is much more dangerous, an abrogation of moral duty, and liable to be much more expensive. Of course, with such totalitarian measures in control, a vast and fierce inspectorial system also has to be provided (which can never police the system effectively). We believe that this cannot be the best use of our national resources.

Even where there is a full and detailed curriculum policy in place, an individual teacher involved in education still should make decisions and carry out activities based upon how they personally see and value educational matters, processes and activities. Decision about all these (including the educational aims, the principles of procedure and other educational principles) is informed by what the teacher values. Together these add up to the teacher's educational philosophy and this will profoundly affect the learner's experiences. The teacher's philosophy and educational values ought to be discussed with learners, but in any case will always be clear to them. Unless teachers have given some thought to what they believe about the educational enterprise, their educational values, and their philosophy, then what they do will (by default) be shaped by events from their own experiences, rather than by intelligent choice from amongst considered alternatives.

The educational matters which teachers decide about and act upon include:

- the educational aims and intentions;
- the teacher's role;
- the nature of learning and what motivates the learner;
- the learner's role;
- the nature of the knowledge to be provided for the learner;
- the structure and order in which the learner will have access to this knowledge;
- how to enable the learner to access and explore this knowledge critically;
- the resources needed;
- the role of assessment;
- the timing of assessment within the overall educational enterprise;
- what counts as evidence of the success of the learner;
- what counts as evidence of the success of the teacher.

For each of the above there is a range of possible choices. What we choose, and what we take into account in order to choose, shows what we value educationally.

However, it is also clear that a wide range of other values will also affect the success of the teaching which is offered. These also need to be recognized and managed by the teacher. Such values are:

- brought with them by learners;
- implicit in medical institutions (Royal Colleges, GMC), and their actions and publications;
- implicit in institutions of higher education and their actions and publications;

- implicit in the individual institution (the hospital Trust) and its policies and practices;
- assumed by the public (in respect of surgery and education) and often shaped by the media;
- embedded in government policy and discernible beneath the surface of government requirements and the language of government documents.

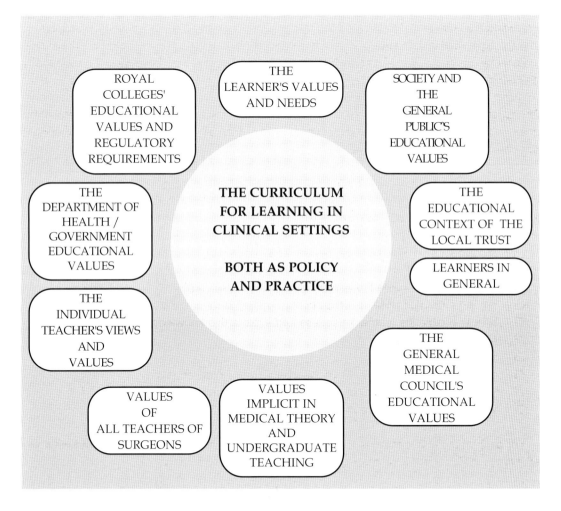

Figure 3:1 Factors and their educational values which shape the curriculum for surgeons in the clinical setting.

See Fish and Coles (forthcoming) for further details about constructing a curriculum and the relationship between the curriculum as a policy and the curriculum in action.

End note

Having looked at the educational practice of the teacher and the significance in it of values and educational principles, we now turn to the central focus of the practising educator. The following chapter therefore, explores why it is that the teacher's most important subject for study is *the learner.*

Chapter 4

Nurturing the learner and supporting learning in the clinical setting

Introduction

Considering the learning context

Nurturing the learner, supporting learning

Introduction

Education engages teachers in seeking to maximize the possibilities for growth of understanding in a learner, and enables learners to make their own best sense out of those possibilities. (It is also true of course that it is possible for understanding to be maximized without a teacher being there at all.) Medical education seeks to promote understanding of how to think like and be like, as well as to act like, a doctor.

Were this book about training, it would focus on the teacher's skills in: questioning and instructing; probing and presenting; scaffolding the learner's response; and giving feedback on the learner's achievements in changing their behaviour. This places the responsibility for most of the action on the teacher's shoulders. But, as we shall see, in education, which is about the learner understanding and so changing or developing their conduct, the teacher's role is to be a support in this enterprise. Here, the teacher's language is much less important than the learner's. Indeed, in some senses, everything about the learner is more important than anything about the teacher!

This chapter then seeks to challenge the assumptions and values that lie under notions that education is about the teacher acquiring and demonstrating a good repertoire of teaching skills because that is what produces desirable educational outcomes. Instead, it seeks to illuminate the importance of maximizing the learner's opportunities for growth of understanding (within which the teacher's skills may play a part but are not the determining factor, and where supportive skills may be more significant than instructional and questioning ones).

Fundamentally, much of this is about a relationship between teacher and learner in which they work together (side by side metaphorically as well as literally) to educational ends that they have negotiated and agreed. This is not quite so much a matter of seeing education as 'learner centred', but rather of seeing it as a collaborative enterprise. In this process, learners need to use spoken language to make sense for themselves of their experiences and of the teacher's exposition. Grundy puts this well, in reference to the teacher's questioning skills, which she sees not as a technical matter but rather as: *'the means by which learning is made meaningful and meaningfulness is monitored'* [italics ours]. She continues:

> 'In this case, the choice of what question to ask becomes a matter of personal judgement, not a matter of skill or strategic decision-making. At another level, however, the asking of questions can be recognized as a fundamental way in which power is both maintained and distributed in a learning situation. In this case, to exercise one's skill in questioning is to exercise control of the learning environment and the learners. To work in a way which distributes power equitably in the learning environment is to adopt an approach to questioning which not only recognizes the importance of judgement, but also the importance of negotiation and symmetry in the discourse of learning.'
>
> (Grundy, 1987, p. 180)

The focus, therefore, is on the learner. The learning environment needs to be shaped to nurture learners as they struggle to make best sense of their experiences and opportunities. The teacher's intentions are about providing the best support for this. In the practice setting this is about developing a safe surgical practicum. Attitudes are also important. The mindset needs to be positive, not negative (both teacher and learner are looking to develop achievement). The starting point must be where the learner currently is, not where teacher thinks, guesses, hopes or mistakenly believes she or he is. What the learner knows (not what they don't know) is what is important. And it is the learner's language (listened to carefully by the teacher) that will provide this information.

The role of the *learner's* talk in learning then is crucial. It enables learners to make meaning for themselves out of the experiences they have had, and provides the teacher with the basis for diagnosis of the learning needs. In medicine, the doctor looks for patterns of health and disease in the patient's physical and mental state, engages in examination and investigation of the patient, and develops with the patient an agreed treatment plan, which is kept under review. In education, the teacher looks for patterns of understanding and achievement in the learner's talk and actions, in order to come to an agreed learning plan in negotiation with the learner, which they both keep under review on a regular basis in the light of the learner's progress. Table 4:1 explores this notion in greater detail.

Table 4:1 Parallels between medical and educational practice.

	MEDICAL PRACTICE	EDUCATIONAL PRACTICE
	Patient centred **The surgeon must:**	**Collaborative with learner** **Teacher and learner together must:**
1.	take history and examine	find out what the learner knows and needs - during educational induction
2.	develop working diagnosis (mainly doctor)	review learner's previous achievements and current needs in the light of what the attachment can offer
3.	carry out investigations	explore current abilities in the clinical setting by review of educational portfolio
4.	review results and formulate treatment plan with patient	agree learning intentions for the attachment and associated assessments and keep under regular review using formative assessment
5.	treat	plan learning opportunities and agree what learner and teacher need to do and carry this out
6.	review treatment	review learning, through learner's reflective talking and writing
7.	treat complications	plan for additional needs as they arise
8.	reconsider whole process	agree that learner should write a review of their achievements during the attachment
9.	record data and outcome (audit)	a) record summative assessment of learner's achievements in the attachment by reference to formative assessments b) record evaluation of the quality of the learning opportunities and the attachment as a whole
10.	discharge patient (requires medical knowledge, knowledge of Trust's systems, processes and record-keeping)	sign off learner (requires: educational understanding of the learner and the nature of learning; knowledge of methods of supporting and assessing learning and methods of educational evaluation; and knowledge of the Trust and the Deanery's educational systems, processes and record-keeping)

The crucial requirement for the teacher then is to understand the learner and the nature of learning, and to know how to support and assess learning. This chapter seeks to provide further enlightenment about these matters, as they relate to learning in clinical settings, by focusing on the learning context, and ways of respecting and nurturing the learner.

Considering the learning context

The context in which learning takes place influences considerably the quality of learning. This is a more complex matter than at first it seems. As well as indicating the physical situation in which learning takes place, the 'context' here refers to the mind of the learner, and all the personal circumstances and entire autobiography that the learner brings to the learning activity. We all have individual preferences about the context and environment in which we most comfortably learn. We are each an expert in our own learning processes and history. A wise educator attends carefully to the learner's in-depth knowledge of these matters. A trainer is less interested in them.

Setting the context for learning

Training often takes little account of the context in which it occurs and sees the learner as passive follower of the teacher's instructions, irrespective of where this is happening, either metaphorically (where the new learning fits within the learner's current understanding and needs) or literally (where the training is taking place). The trainer shows relatively little interest in the learner, seeks a neutral territory in which to work, scaffolds the learner's understanding, by providing language which creates the world into which the learner enters, and gives the learner feedback about success.

This metaphor comes from Bruner (but was first used by Vygotski). Bruner contended that in the 'act of interacting' between people, teachers 'create the world into which the child enters'. 'Scaffolding' is the process of transferring skills from teacher to learner, whereby an adult supports a child in learning a new task and gradually withdraws control as the child gains mastery. The idea of teacher providing learner with a scaffolding framework (with its temporarily constructed parallel poles which are bolted together in the air to form both the bases for flooring planks to stand on and open spaces within which to work), promotes a view of learning as a process of constructing new ideas based on current or past knowledge. It is 'a constructionist' view of education, and arose in relation to teaching in schools.

The metaphors used to present these ideas give a strong clue to their underlying values. In this version of scaffolding, the teacher provides the overall shape of how to do something, which the learner conforms to. There is a strong sense of the teacher as the master builder. It has to be asked whether this does justice to the nature of learning, as educators understand it and learners know it. There is an implication in this constructionist view that learning can be 'mastered', that learners all learn in the same way, and that learning is about progressing through levels, which are incremental, pre-determined, even-paced and can be simply shaped by the teacher. There is also an underlying assumption that what teacher 'transmits' will automatically be received intact by the learner. This view of the nature of learning is flawed, as even the briefest consideration of one's own learning patterns will demonstrate. We all learn by fits and starts not by walking a smooth incremental path, and our most exciting and creative learning occurs when the goals are *not* all pre-determined. We have preferences for how to learn and we prefer different learning environments (some wanting silence, some wanting music as a background, for example). The notion of teaching as being about 'transmitting what the teacher knows', which the learner simply receives and caches in the memory, is also highly problematic, and takes no account of what generations of research in education have taught us about teaching and learning, the mind and the memory.

Learners must make sense *for themselves* of learning situations and learning opportunities, because when teacher transmits new knowledge to learners, they have as individuals to re-interpret it on the basis of what they already know. This means that in the most successful teaching:

❐   the emphasis is on the activities, language and meaning-making of the learner;
❐   the quality of the teaching/learning interaction is far more dependent on the meaning-making of the learner than on the transmission skills of the teacher;
❐   at minimum, if scaffolding is to be used, it is constructed between learner and teacher, not given by teacher through teacher's questions and instruction;
❐   for every learner a slightly different interpretation is placed on the teacher's words;
❐   learners need the chance to formulate and check out the sense they make of new topics;
❐   teachers need to know what sense learners are making of what they offer, rather than assuming that they know;
❐   this also values and respects what the learner brings to the learning.

No one can learn for another. Since knowledge can only be made sense of by individual learners who need at best to be actively engaged, clearly, education needs to be based on a partnership between teachers and learners, in which the responsibility for selecting and organizing the learning activities is shared in a mutually supportive environment which will inevitably be non-discriminatory in respect of all politically correct matters.

Thus, the curriculum becomes negotiated; teachers become experts in facilitating learning, in guiding learners to re-invent knowledge and in enriching their meaning-making; and learners begin to take control of their learning, become experts in recognizing learning opportunities and pro-active in working on them, and can engage in self-assessment. How then might these notions be played out in the clinical setting?

The clinical setting as a context for learning

For doctors and surgeons, the reality of learning within the clinical setting has until now involved the learner in picking up within each attachment, whenever, and from wherever possible, a series of pieces of wisdom about procedures, processes and factual knowledge related to generic medical knowledge and the surgical specialty. As Eraut and du Boulay, (2000), pointed out, this is too haphazard to ensure sound education. This is particularly true given the constraints on time which have become typical of medical practice in Britain in the 21st Century.

SHOs in surgical practice, as we noted in passing in Chapter 1, have been characterized as engaging mainly in 'magpie' learning (Brigley, *et al*, 2003). The metaphor is apt in that it highlights the lack of system and rigour involved, and pictures learners as scurrying around the clinical setting with a predatory eye out for what they *take to be* the best (or most easily accessed) jewels of wisdom, which they seize wholesale as valuable acquisitions, and rush off to store in random order in the bottom of their nest, against the day when they might come in handy, but perhaps without analyzing or having any idea why they are valuable. This is how the constructionst view of teaching and learning has evolved in the clinical setting. The teacher assumes that the provision of opportunity to experience practice, and the accompanying instructions and questions from the teacher, will scaffold learning sufficiently to ensure that the 'correct message' is gained so that specific learning can be mastered. But the learner rarely has the opportunity of sharing and checking out the appropriateness of the meaning they have made of the opportunity. The context for learning here lacks structure within the learner's head, within the teacher's mind, and within the physical context.

The arenas from which such jewels are seized (and in which more rigorous education now needs to take place) are of four kinds:

1. Self-directed learning (where the learner uses a range of published resources to gain information to support planned clinical activity in response to service needs and to prepare for examination answers on guessed-at topics).

2. Formal teaching in theatre, ward and clinic (where the learner receives from a more senior clinician pre-planned instruction and scheduled opportunities for practising clinical processes and procedures, the choice of topic being whatever suits the clinical need of the time).

3. Informal (unplanned) teaching in theatre, ward and clinic (where the eventualities of the service are utilized entirely opportunistically by teachers and/or learners).

4. Informal occasions in the interstices of practice (in corridors, between cases, in the tea room) when talking turns to something the learner finds educational (and in which some of the most profound and formative thoughts and ideas are generated).

Such activity, however, barely merits the term postgraduate education, in that it is mainly opportunistic, remains largely unplanned, and leaves learners to piece it all together as best they can but without checking whether they can, and without providing any means for connecting this to other understanding within the learners' minds. Further, it omits (or leaves tacit and therefore largely unattended to) some important and key elements that have come to be understood as central to the successful learning process. These are:

1. the need for learners to have some choice about their preferred ways of learning and not be expected to receive knowledge as if it were a product to be delivered by the teacher to the learner (since learners learn at different rates and in different ways);

2. the need for learners to link their new knowledge to what was known previously (so that adjustments are thoughtfully made to their previous knowledge as well as recognition being given to recent acquisitions);

3. the need to make overall sense of the territory and establish links and connections between various areas of newly gained knowledge (because teachers offer individual pieces of knowledge and do not automatically take responsibility for putting them into the wider context for the learner);

4. the need to know which jewels are worth seizing, how to prioritize them, and why (because they are all offered separately as if of equal value, when in fact some are more important than others);

5. the need to understand the underlying structure of the knowledge used in clinical practice in order to be able to make cohesive those randomly picked up elements, and to be sure that some bits have not simply been missed out because their availability is not readily apparent to the roving scavenger (because individual surgical teachers may not take responsibility for structure, continuity and balance of the whole educational curriculum if they offer only their particular piece of it);

6. the need for learners to treat knowledge not as a product to be handed from the teacher to the learner and placed in store, but as something they use and make their own by putting it into their own language, thus turning their new knowledge into understanding (because knowing something as a fact is very different from coming to understand it and its implications).

For these reasons, the learner needs to have access to, or to have considered the following:

1. an overall map of the territory to be learnt: this is not simply a list of things to be learnt (a syllabus), but at minimum, a map of the knowledge base, constructed between key teacher and learner, showing key relationships, or at best, a whole properly constructed curriculum to which teachers and learners are working, and which both parties use to ensure coherence and continuity, thus providing a necessary rigour and system to shape the learning;

2. understanding of how they best learn the various sorts of knowledge necessary;

3.   understanding that learning is about learners each constructing their own meaning from the resources offered to them and checking this with the teacher (because learning involves a conversation between teacher and learner, rather than a monologue from the teacher);

4.   knowledge of the resources available to them for the purpose of learning on the particular attachment and what these are most appropriate for.

The induction process should have attended at a formal level to these, but they need to be revisited regularly during the attachment, and they also need to be understood by all those who will act as a resource for the learner in the clinical setting throughout the programme. This includes all the professionals with whom the learner comes into contact.

By this means a safe environment will be established in which the learner can be properly nurtured whilst being exposed to the full panoply of experience in real practice. In the educational provision of other professions, this safe environment is often referred to as a 'safe practicum', following the ideas of Schön.

The need for a safe clinical practicum for learning surgery

Almost twenty years ago, in the context of professional education generally, Schön defined and recommended the establishment within each profession of 'a setting designed for the task of learning a [professional] practice.' He argued that a safe practicum can be established, 'in a context that approximates a practice world [where] students learn by doing, although their doing often falls short of real-world work....' The practicum 'is a virtual world, relatively free of the pressures, distractions and risk of the real one to which, nevertheless, it refers' (Schön, 1987, p. 37). The practicum is where the learner is initiated into being a member of a community of practice and 'tries out' practice within the community, taking responsibility in this.

We like this idea of a group of like-minded learners being and working together, and taking joint learning responsibilities for each other's development (see also Wenger, 1999). It simulates the best of what happens (or should happen) in the clinical setting. We recognize however, that Schön's definition was designed for an undergraduate setting and we believe that it is insufficiently developed for use in the clinical setting, where postgraduate doctors take on *full* personal responsibility for the care of patients at the same time as being a trainee.

We have already argued that apprenticeship falls short as a definition of relationships and activities of postgraduate learners (see Chapter 1). We offer in its place, as a development of Schön's idea, the term 'clinical practicum' as more suitable to describe the setting for postgraduate learning in medicine. We define clinical practicum as a clinical environment (including the full clinical team) which has been prepared for the task of facilitating the education of trainees as they practise surgery within a real live setting. Here, they have direct responsibilities for both patient care and their own postgraduate development, which will be facilitated by their teachers. Surgery involves performing invasive actions on patients as part of their treatment. Surgical learners need careful support if they are to operate safely on patients and at the same time learn from this process. Such support (from all the team) must be designed to enable the learner to take as much control as possible, not only of the operation, but also of the educational spin-off from doing it. To foster this approach, the team need to use educational processes designed to achieve these ends. The understanding out of which they develop these is gained from a consideration of the nature of learning as we illustrate it in the rest of this chapter.

A safe clinical practicum therefore, is where the environment is set to provide the best care of patients, whilst ensuring a sympathetic educational context for the learner and which also attends to the protection of the teacher. We would argue that this environment is urgently needed, in order to minimize the risks involved in real life clinical service by attending to the development of the surgeons of the future, as a central requirement for providing for the surgical needs of the nation.

It is crucial to remember too, that this safe clinical practicum for learning surgeons is part of, and related to, a much larger learning community. The hospital Trust has a responsibility to nurture such a learning environment and will be called to account for the quality of it at times of external review of its educational facilities.

What we are beginning to see is that learning is essentially collaborative. Within this collaborative approach, the nurturing context is an important element. Most people would agree with this, but in reality it is sadly easy for the wrong signals to be flagged to a learner from the very start of the attachment, as the following shows.

Two examples of setting the context and structuring education

We offer the following two brief related examples as a means of illustrating the significance of context in educational activities. The first shows how difficult it still is to give substance and gravitas to the importance of meeting learners and finding out about them at the beginning of a post. The second is an example of how a properly supportive, collaborative and nurturing context can be set at the beginning of an attachment by the development and agreement between teachers and learners of a learning contract.

Example one: induction

Educational induction is a new process for surgeons, and it offers us a good example of the importance of the context for learning, and of how the learner is drawn to make assumptions about the educational environment of the whole attachment. Every induction occasion provides the learner with a foreshadowing of how they will be seen and treated, and of the values which are accorded to the educational process they hope to engage in. Being placed at the very start of a new post, induction and how it is handled will be sharply observed by learners. The values and signposts given out by how induction is handled are embedded in the very structure of induction, as the following Table 4:2 shows.

Table 4:2 Types of induction for SHOs in surgery.

| | TRUST | DEPARTMENTAL | | SPECIALTY TRAINING PROGRAMME | |
	Managerial	Managerial	Educational	Managerial	Educational
Requirement	MANDATORY	MANDATORY	NOT MANDATORY	NOT MANDATORY	NOT MANDATORY
Reason	• To comply with national requirements • To ensure delivery of information on a range of non-clinical matters • Trust accreditation performance will be affected by it	• To comply with Trust requirements • To ensure delivery of organisational information • To serve the needs of a potential disciplinary/ risk process	• To set educational framework • To comply with Deanery requirements	• To know what to do and what is expected of them contractually	• To know what to do and what is expected of them educationally
Interested parties	Chief Executive & Medical Director Clinical Director DOH	Chief Executive & Medical Director Clinical Director Lead Clinician Directorate manager	Specialty Tutor BST Committee Individual consultants	Programme Director	Programme Director
Process	Fixed sessions at the beginning of a post as an alternative to clinical activity	Fixed sessions at the beginning of a post as alternative to clinical activity	Fixed into the department's educational programme	Not a fixed meeting Info by post Information on one to one by Programme Director	Not a fixed meeting Info by post Information on one to one by Programme Director
Who manages?	Manager with fixed sessions	Manager with fixed sessions	Consultant with no fixed sessions	Programme Director: no fixed sessions	Programme Director: no fixed sessions
SHO responsibilities	Required to attend	Required to attend	Invited to attend	Invited to attend	Invited to attend

It is clear from the above that the educational aspects of induction are not yet privileged, in the way that Trust level induction is, are not a requirement of either the teacher or the learner, and can easily degenerate into a postal exercise at best and at worst may not happen at all. By comparison, there are now some Trusts in which surgeons are not only meeting learners personally, but are offering their own CV to those with whom they are going to work, are

Table 4:3 An agenda for the educational induction of SHOs in surgery.

Exploring the learner's starting points

Key agenda items in clarifying the intentions of the attachment

- Check that the learner has and has read any relevant curriculum papers
- Review professional values and educational values
- Establish the learner's level of experience
- Establish the learner's preferred and best ways of learning in clinical settings
- Reveal the key specialisms that this attachment can offer the learner
- Consider the teacher's preferred ways of bringing education and service togther
- Identify main elements of the syllabus which the attachment will focus on
- Ensure understanding of the content and processes of the portfolio
- Ensure understanding of the triggered assessments
- Agree and document the intentions for the attachment

exploring with the learner their starting points and their educational needs for the attachment, and are setting up joint agreements about ways forward. (We acknowledge that the use of consultant CVs at induction was first developed by Lester Sher.) Table 4:3 offers the kind of agenda now being used in the best educational induction meeting.

Learning surgeons are now beginning to attend these discussions with:

- ❏ a clear list of their professional values;
- ❏ an analysis of their surgical/clinical experience to date;
- ❏ an analysis of their learning needs for this attachment (so far as they can see them);
- ❏ some notes on how they see themselves as a learner; and
- ❏ a brief CV.

All these are placed in the introductory section of their learning portfolio for the attachment.

Example two: agreeing a learning contract

A learning contract (a negotiated learning plan) indicates the commitments of the parties to the study involved. Such contracts:

- ❏ help to clarify roles;
- ❏ establish ownership;
- ❏ improve the quality of learning by clarifying learning intentions;
- ❏ establish the processes of and for collaboration;
- ❏ establish the character of the learning environment and group;

❒ enable all parties to be explicit about their assumptions about the learning that will take place;

❒ provide (some of the) criteria for an evaluation of the educational enterprise.

Processes in setting up a contract include:

❒ recognizing the scope of the bargaining area and the range of negotiation possible;
❒ valuing everyone involved;
❒ identifying learning intentions;
❒ the teacher listening more than talking;
❒ being neutral and factual;
❒ actively seeking mutual acceptability;
❒ each knowing the concessions they can make;
❒ being willing to be innovative;
❒ formalizing the result in writing.

The development of a learning contract with these kinds of characteristics, during an educational induction process, has a great deal to tell learners about how they are valued, how they can learn, the collaborative nature of such learning, and above all, the view of education held and its importance in the post. A learning contract establishes a mindset in both teacher and learner. This will quickly become eroded if it is not regularly revisited, renegotiated and readjusted. It is important that it does not focus the learner on one teacher, because there are many resources for learning in the clinical setting.

Professionals as members of a range of learning communities

Professionals are members of a range of professional communities, in each of which the professional has responsibilities to his/her fellows. This makes professional practice (and the learning of that practice) a social and collaborative enterprise. Such professional communities include the community of the workplace, of one's specialist knowledge, of one's professional body, and of professions generally.

This of course means that there are more resources to support learning in both the clinical setting and the learner's wider professional context, than was assumed in traditional approaches to clinical teaching described in Chapter 1. Figure 4:1 sets out the main sources of help for learners as they attempt to make sense of their experiences and learning opportunities.

Learning in a community of practice

Wenger, (1999), offers us some important processes for learning in communities of practice. These include (which learning surgeons will need to explore within their Trust and department):

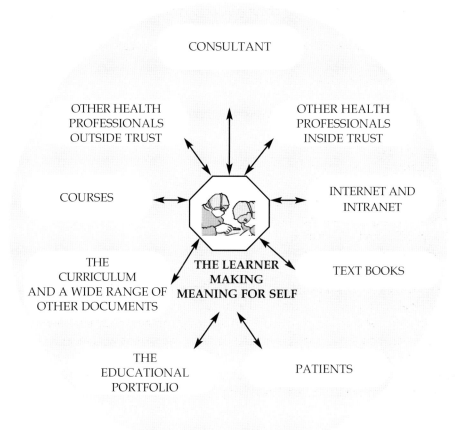

Figure 4:1 The resources available for learners in clinical settings.

1. evolving forms of mutual engagement: discovering how to engage, what helps, what hinders, developing mutual relationships; defining identities, establishing who is who, who is good at what, who knows what, and who is easy or hard to get along with;

2. understanding and tuning their enterprise: aligning their engagement with that of the Trust, learning to become and hold each other accountable to it, struggling to define what the enterprise is all about;

3. developing their repertoire, styles and discourses: renegotiating the meaning and recognizing the importance of various elements, recalling events, inventing new terms, creating and breaking routines.

These three dimensions of learning, he argues, are interdependent and interlocked into a tight system. He also usefully discusses a range of social perspectives on learning, and makes the following key points. Learning:

- ❐ is inherent in human nature;
- ❐ is first and foremost the ability to negotiate new meanings;
- ❐ is fundamentally experiential and social;
- ❐ transforms our identities;
- ❐ helps build personal histories in relation to the social histories of our communities, in a process of individual and collective 'becoming';
- ❐ means dealing with boundaries (creates bridges and parameters);
- ❐ depends on negotiating power relationships;
- ❐ depends on opportunities to contribute actively to the practices of the communities that we value and that value us;
- ❐ is a matter of the imagination (depends on the ability to put oneself in the place of others);
- ❐ involves an inter-play between the local and the global.

(See Wenger, 1999, pp. 226-228)

Nurturing the learner, supporting learning

Educational understanding involves recognizing fundamental principles for nurturing the learner. These include an understanding that good learning should:

- ❐ be conducted in a sheltered and supportive context;
- ❐ be transformative (in that it changes understanding and by this means changes conduct);
- ❐ be active and interactive;
- ❐ be intrinsically motivating;
- ❐ be life-long;
- ❐ take place within the context of nurturing relationships;
- ❐ be transacted through rich communications;
- ❐ recognize that the role of the learner's talk is central.

(See Collins, Harkin and Nind, 2002; and Fish, 2005)

This section looks at some of these issues in more detail.

Ways of drawing the learner into communities of practice

Teachers need to recognize and to take account of the complexities and subtleties, the taken-for-granted elements of everyday life, in order to prepare professionals for these. This demands the ability to articulate the tacit as well as the overt elements of their own practice, and their professionalism. They need to enable practitioners to develop critical perspectives on them so that they are aware of how the individual practice of one community relates to the practice of the wider professional community, and are able to reconsider and even redesign their practice and the practice of their profession. The following table sets out the issues about drawing the learner to move from the specifics of one attachment to the wider issues of professional practice.

Table 4:4 The wider issues of professional practice.

Practice on an individual attachment and with individual patients can:		
• emphasize the practical	but	how does this relate to the visions and wider views of professional work, which also need attention?
• focus on the specific (is highly contextualized)	but	of what generalizable value is this?
• be idiosyncratic	but	why then should we pay attention to it?
• offer learners opportunities to observe great expertise in good practitioners, some of which is deeply embedded in practice and invisible	so	how can we give learners access to this?

It is the case, then, that particular clinical experience must induct learners into the profession but that such experience must transfer to other places and later times; that individual clinical experiences must be understood as part of a broad social practice and its sets of conflicting traditions; that access to broader understanding involves reviewing the assumptions that underlie the provision of clinical practice; that unearthing these assumptions, beliefs and values is a matter of learning to theorize from practice. (We acknowledge that these ideas were first expressed orally by Professor Mike Golby).

In fostering learning through clinical practice, it is important to consider:

❑ the educational aims of the clinical experience;
❑ the kind of experience it actually is and how it can be used educationally;
❑ the kind of learning and teaching involved;
❑ the ability to theorize practice;
❑ the role of assessment in that learning;
❑ how that individual learning experience relates to becoming a professional.

All this is more efficacious if the entire team share such an agenda and subscribe to the key principles of collaborative learning.

Engaging the learner in collaborative learning

Collaboration is more than co-operation (working to a common end). It involves co-operation, pooling ideas, working across boundaries, sharing goals, and the readiness of peers to grant and accept authority. It is growth-oriented teaching. It is very powerful. It achieves more for learners than does competitiveness. It is interested in educational processes as well as products.

Collaborative learning:

- [ ] increases the complexity of thinking;
- [ ] enables the acceptance of other/wider ideas;
- [ ] enriches ideas;
- [ ] increases motivation;
- [ ] brings a community together;
- [ ] calls forth from learners levels of ingenuity and inventiveness that they didn't know they possessed;
- [ ] brings support and feedback for learners;
- [ ] improves understanding via discussion and controversy;
- [ ] generates energy and more active participation;
- [ ] can transform thinking and living;
- [ ] has social and affective (emotional) benefits;
- [ ] leads to longer-term retention of ideas.

The teacher also needs to be able to handle reflection, dialogue and argument amongst learners. This means that the teacher will take risks, because much of this will change the power relationships. Teachers and learners are therefore best supported in learning communities.

The importance of nurturing the learner's language

We said at the start of this chapter that the learner's language is particularly important. Communicating with others is a complex process. Professional conversation and/or spoken and written reflection provides learners with an opportunity to re-invent the knowledge they have gained and to make sense of it in their own terms. We - every one of us - are meaning-makers. Communicating with others involves:

- [ ] intending to inform/request/persuade them;
- [ ] having in mind an idea, (event, action) that we intend that someone else should understand.

Our words and ideas spring from a personal model of the world which we each have, and which has been developed through our individual life experiences. This means that no one else has exactly the same mental model as we do. Also, because words have to be selected and arranged in sequence, even when our listener is able to form the same ideas as we have, we cannot transmit ours to him directly and simultaneously as they arise. (Speech lags behind thought.) Further, the public and general words we use do not always fit perfectly our private and personal thoughts. It is simply not possible, therefore, to convey the ideas that we have in mind in a form that does full justice to their simultaneous complexity and specificity.

Of course, in normal conversation all our past experience of language and the world to which it refers, and of our shared culture (to the extent that it *is* shared), is sufficiently similar to enable us to share a good basis for understanding. And when we are not clear, we have strategies for seeking clarification. Indeed, in a conversation (which is a kind of improvisation) where meaning is jointly construed, we can modify and amplify our ideas and their expression in the light of feedback. But where the participants in a conversation come from different cultural backgrounds, or where they differ considerably in level of experience and knowledge, the possibility of misunderstanding is ever present.

Teacher and learner therefore need to take care that the meanings constructed between them do not become increasingly divergent.

For this reason, the teacher needs to:

❏   listen carefully to what the learner says;
❏   try to understand it from the learner's view-point;
❏   take the learner's meanings as the basis for what s/he says next;
❏   use vocabulary and syntax (word order) which the learner understands.

Conversation between teacher and learner therefore needs to be treated as a collaborative enterprise. This is why the teacher who is merely a transmitter of knowledge often does not succeed in getting the knowledge over to learners. It is not possible, by telling, to cause learners to have the knowledge that is in the mind of the teacher. Indeed, knowledge cannot be transmitted, but has to be constructed afresh by each individual on the basis of what is already known to him/her, and by means of strategies s/he has developed in life. This is a *re-constructionist* view of education, which works on the following tenets.

❏   For every learner a slightly different interpretation is placed on the teacher's words.
❏   Learners need the chance to formulate and check out the sense they make of new topics.
❏   Teachers too, need to know what sense learners are making of what they offer.
❏   This also values what the learner brings to the learning.

(See Wells, 1986/2002)

Nurturing the learner, supporting learning

No one can learn for (on behalf of) another person. At best we can:

- ❑ set up learning situations which encourage and motivate learning;
- ❑ engage learners in exploring their understanding (see how they construct in their minds the learning provided) and then help them to reshape it;
- ❑ listen to their language and hear what sense they have made of the learning they have engaged in;
- ❑ attend positively to the self-image of the learner;
- ❑ help learners to develop learning strategies that they are comfortable with;
- ❑ enable them to reflect systematically and in detail on their practice;
- ❑ encourage them to begin to investigate their own practice;
- ❑ encourage them to engage in self-assessment;
- ❑ offer them a model of all these in the very way we conduct ourselves.

In these terms, teaching has been recast from being merely instruction and involves:

- ❑ valuing what the learner has to offer;
- ❑ seeing mistakes as a positive contribution to learning;
- ❑ taking risks;
- ❑ being imaginative (putting yourself in the learner's place);
- ❑ being prevenient (going ahead to prepare the way);
- ❑ valuing the journey (for learners) as much as their arrival;
- ❑ offering clear debriefing about the learning - via a professional conversation;
- ❑ educating - never just training.

We can improve learning: by studying the learner; by ensuring that we know the learner and have established good human relationships with him or her as a first priority; by starting where the learner is and taking account of what he or she already knows; by looking always for evidence to challenge our previous assumptions about the learner; by shaping what we teach to the character, characteristics and ability level of the learner; by involving learners actively and deeply in their own education; by emphasizing the learner's positive achievements, and by engaging the learner in co-operation with others, thus developing a learning community.

Much learning in the clinical setting depends upon well-disciplined reflection on the experiences provided and the learning opportunities available. Accordingly, the following chapter looks in detail at the processes involved in reflection.

Chapter 5

Reflection: an essential means of learning in clinical settings

Introduction

Reflection: an overview
A range of roles for reflection
A range of topics to focus on and reasons for reflection
The key means of engaging in reflection

Exploring reflection in professional education
Some definitions of reflection
Some defining characteristics of reflective practice
Some historical perspectives

What surgeons might reflect on and how they might do so
Exploring holistic surgical practice through reflection
Some key processes for reflecting on practice

Writing reflectively: some starting points
The key differences between talking and writing reflectively
The key characteristics of reflective writing
Some suggestions for refining reflective writing

End note

Introduction

Having an experience is not the same as understanding its meaning. There is far more to a clinical event than is visible on its surface. Reflection is a very important process which enables a learner to make meaning out of experience (making the invisible visible), and which allows the teacher to ensure that the fullest and most appropriate learning has been gained from it. Reflection points up the significance of a key event in the clinical setting on which there is no time to dwell fully within the on-going speed of practice, and triggers a depth of understanding of it that could never be built and explored during the heat of action.

Reflection is particularly useful for learning surgeons, helping them to enrich their practical knowledge from selected learning opportunities. It places understanding their practice (and thus being able to refine, and develop or change it) as central to their educational agenda. As a key means of unearthing all that lies beneath the visible surface of practice, reflection is about *generating knowledge* out of practice. It enables learners to consider critically and develop those forces that drive their practice, and it ultimately allows them to be assessed in a more holistic way than merely focusing on visible skills would permit. Now that learners' time in the practice setting has been reduced by the prevailing conditions of the 21st Century, reflection is set to become an indispensable part of surgical education.

For those not yet fully familiar with reflective practice, this chapter provides an overview of it and establishes the foundations that learning surgeons and their teachers need, in order to develop and assess surgical practice, as illustrated throughout most of Part two.

Reflection: an overview

This first section sets the scene by explaining the context which gives rise to different ways of seeing reflection, looking at the range of subjects on which reflection can usefully be focused and the reasons for engaging in it, and noting the variety of formats in which it can occur.

A range of roles for reflection

As we have already seen in Chapter 3, learning in all cases implies change, but there are different schools of thought about the *kind* of change that is desirable. With these various views come different versions of reflection (its purpose, value and role in learning, and in providing evidence of learning).

Trainers, seeking to change behaviour in ways that are visible and measurable, will at best require reflection merely to offer an endorsement of the new or changed activity, and at worst will deny reflection any significance at all. Training, as we have shown, depends specifically on feedback during the process. Such feedback is traditionally given initially by teacher to learner, until the teacher's model of how to do it is taken up by the learner. Feedback contains critique and is rarely exploratory in spirit, but it can lead the learner ultimately to engage in self-reflection, albeit narrowly focused (see Chapter 4). By contrast, those seeking to change or develop a learner's understanding, cultivate a learner's mind, and/or emancipate a learner to a point of independence from the teacher, will actually need to draw the learner to reflect, and will see it as a vital educational process and an integral part of learning. Indeed, 'an emancipatory curriculum entails a reciprocal relationship between self-reflection and action' (Grundy, 1987, p. 19).

Within education, reflection is not a bolt-on optional extra. It comes as part of the curriculum. It can specifically enable meaning to be made out of an experience, and enhance the learning that can emerge from it. In particular, it is a key process in education in clinical settings, and thus is an integral part of 'learning to practise'. It balances the training element (which develops pure skills) by attending to the thinking and knowing that needs to underlie them in real clinical activities if the practice is to be truly and consciously intelligent. That is why reflection has been taken up as significant by so many professions. The literature of teaching, nursing, occupational therapy, physiotherapy and a wide range of other professions related to medicine, has long been full of serious contributions to this field through which these professions learn from and develop each other.

A range of topics to focus on and reasons for reflection

Reflection on practice is a means of getting more out of the experiences available, and so it is particularly relevant now that learners' opportunities for engaging in surgical practice have become fewer, and the years in training are being reduced. It enables a practitioner to explore a wide range of topics, as follows.

Reflection enables learners to:

- explore, make sense of, and thus understand more fully their current experiences, actions and events;
- contextualize these current experiences and relate them critically to other relevant theory and practice;
- extend their current competence in clinical practice;
- recognize new challenges to work on, in clinical practice;
- appreciate the subtleties of clinical practice;
- connect particular practice experiences, events and activities to wider ideas and ideals of practice across their profession;
- develop a personal vision of clinical practice;
- provide evidence of growing insight and progress in understanding;
- crystallize and summarize progress at the end of various stages of learning.

But all this occurs only under certain conditions, and only when the purpose of reflection is itself educational, as opposed to concerned with health care management or therapeutic relief (see Proctor, 1986).

As they learn their practice, surgeons daily engage in, or are party to, a wide range of activities in the clinical setting. These include: having a particular experience, being involved in an event, carrying out an action, learning or practising a skill or skills. But their practice is holistic. These things all happen together, happen fast and fluently, and many of the elements involved are invisible, and so *undergoing* these activities, even being able to enact and re-enact them, is not the same as *understanding* them. Indeed, it would be possible to go through many of them, without engaging the mind at all, rather as we sometimes find when we have driven somewhere on auto-pilot not consciously noticing the detail of the route because our mind has been elsewhere. It is possible to have the experience but to fail to make meaning out of it, not to notice the finer points of it (not recognizing the principles that can be drawn from it; not making links between it and other relevant occurrences or previous learning; not seeing or not sorting out and considering the salient elements in it).

Considerably more value will be extracted from clinical practice, where reflection enables the learner to focus intelligently upon it in order to make meaning out of it (understand it). In the early stages especially, this needs to be shared and validated by reference to the experience of more senior practitioners. It should be remembered that learners do not always make the same profound sense out of something that experts have long seen as having significant features. Indeed, while one part of education is about encouraging learners to recognize and share their visions of their current achievements, another part is about enabling them to see more and differently than they would if left alone, and to help them tease out meanings and significances that they would otherwise miss. This is why reflection needs to be shared by learners with both teachers and peers.

There are other reasons too for engaging in reflection as part of learning in clinical settings. As members of a profession, we work with and for vulnerable people. This brings special responsibilities. For the sake of one's patients, therefore, there is a need to:

- ❐ be able to dig one's theories and values out from under one's practice, in order to examine, explore and even challenge them (or to recognize that one's practice doesn't match up to one's theories and values);
- ❐ be a seeker rather than a knower;
- ❐ recognize one's uncertainties and to use them as growing-points;
- ❐ step back and take a long view of oneself and one's practice;
- ❐ explore the qualities of professionalism and consider oneself against them. (These include looking at the kind of person one is: one's virtues, dispositions, habits of mind, shortcomings, capacities, values, beliefs, theories, ideas, attitudes, commitments, ideals, principles, feelings, understandings, imagination, criticality.)

The key means of engaging in reflection

There are many formats or models and guidelines that offer ways of shaping attempts at reflection, but, as other professions have already found, they are only useful in the early stages while practitioners find their own voice. In general, the key means of engaging in reflection are talking and writing. It is essentially dialogic. It thrives on interaction. It develops through being shared and being worked over and refined. That is why talking something through reflectively will help, and why written dialogue through e-mails is beginning to support learners in F2 programmes. Beyond this, too, there is no substitute for producing and refining an extended piece of writing from time to time, because it reveals more as you go along, and anyone can do it. The most difficult thing is starting; once professionals have begun this process, they rarely abandon it.

This chapter provides an overview of reflection, looks at the kind of learning opportunities that can be enhanced by reflection and at the processes involved.

Exploring reflection in professional education

Some definitions of reflection

There is no one simple definition of reflection that does full justice to its nature. However, we can make some general points, which are likely to hold good in all circumstances. For example, we would want to say that in principle, reflection is certainly not the same as meditation, nor is it a quick chat about what has happened to us, nor a collegiate discussion about policy and practice within a department. Rather, we would argue the following, which emphasizes the holistic nature of practice.

Reflection is about:

- seeking to uncover rigorously and understand and articulate the relationship between one's visions, values and beliefs, and one's thought, knowledge and action, in reference to specific examples of one's own practice;
- having an exploratory cast of mind, that is both critical and meticulous;
- processes which crucially include contextualizing one's practice, viewing and investigating it critically, and exploring open-mindedly how it relates to wider understandings of that practice and the practice of one's profession;
- understanding our practice better, and thus being motivated and committed to improving it, and thereby being equipped to go about such improvement.

In that sense, reflective practice is a special kind of practice, which involves systematic critical enquiry into one's professional work and one's relationship to it. This approach to practice is also known by its Aristotelian term *praxis*, which as we shall see, is about morally informed action, or action shaped by critical consideration of its ends and means. This involves standing back from that practice (and ourselves as part of that practice) and viewing as an observer might, both that practice and our beliefs, assumptions, expectations, feelings, attitudes and values as they impact on our practice. Indeed, it means standing outside the practice of one's profession as a whole and its traditions, and seeing it anew. Grundy makes this point well when she says that there is a tendency in those who engage in the risky domain of human action:

'... to be guided in judgements about that action by an interpretation of the meaning of the situation which is constrained by traditional meanings.... The problem is to act in ways that are not already pre-determined by habitual practice.'

Going on to quote Arendt's work she adds:

'Action which proceeds from judgement-making is a more authentic form of human endeavour than rule-generating or rule-following behaviour.'

(Grundy, 1987, p. 175)

Given the current climate, a particularly useful focus for individual surgical practitioners might be determining, within their own practice, which actions are properly rule-governed and which are not. Serious practical enquiry into their own work would equip them with the ability (when needed on the spot):

❑   to articulate the arguments for maintaining control over their clinical thought and action (which is always at risk from risk management); and

❑   to share powerful and persuasive evidence of the importance of the discretionary decisions and judgements.

It should be noted however, that we are not saying that reflection is something that can be carried out in depth on all one's practice all the time. A serious piece of reflection deserves time and attention and should be carefully chosen. More value is likely to emerge from homing in upon a few incidents a month than will come from working in less depth on a greater number. It is, however, worth adopting a mindset which is always alert to finding a suitable aspect of practice to enquire into. The choice of topic/event should be made for its likely educational impact in respect of one's *own* practice (though reflection upon practical examples of habits and rituals has important things to teach us too). In that sense, reflective practice will probably not coincide with talking through an adverse medical incident for medico-legal purposes, and it is unlikely to be the same activity as discussion of an event for the purposes of risk management. However, the ability to present evidence of regular inquiry into one's own practice in order to develop it, would in any discussion of a problematic legal or risk management situation, provide significant empirical proof of one's on-going concern for good practice.

Some defining characteristics of reflective practice

What more can we say then about reflection, beyond the level of principle? It is possible to offer a range of characteristics which are typical of engagement in reflective practice. Moon offers a range of features, some of which we have summarized as follows.

❑   The subject matter is likely to be (we would say should be) one's own practice and its particular context.

❑   Reflection may be on everyday events, or on the conditions that shape action and thought.

❑   Reflection may focus on an on-going experience or a one-off event.

❑   It is likely to be triggered by uncertainty about something in the mind of the practitioner.

❑   It will engage with moral and ethical content (professional work being morally centred).

❑   It will be precipitated by questions/tasks/personal considerations/problematic issues, to which there is no *simple* solution.

❑   It will have strongly critical elements.

❑   Its endpoint is the attainment of better understanding in the context of improving practice generally.

❑   It is not just about thinking, but articulating that thinking in spoken or written form and as a result being able to extend, refine and develop it.

❑   It is enhanced when shared with others.

(See Moon, 1999, p. 64-65)

We believe that other activities, attributes and characteristics are as follows. Reflective practice:

- ☐ involves a careful consideration of one's own practice through systematic critical enquiry;
- ☐ involves investigating practice from as many points of view as possible;
- ☐ creates opportunities for professional growth and development, because it aims at better understanding of practice;
- ☐ involves standing back from practice and offers the possibility of thinking about it from outside the existing traditions or established patterns of practice;
- ☐ is about reviewing (re-viewing) practice in all its aspects;
- ☐ is about practitioners coming to an understanding of their actions, their espoused theories and theories-in-use;
- ☐ includes moral questions about the worthwhile nature of activities themselves, and thus attends to ends as well as means;
- ☐ engages us in critical thinking;
- ☐ does not replace one set of dogmas with another;
- ☐ does not come in pre-determined forms;
- ☐ is a particularly intimate mode of educational research;
- ☐ is a concept eternally being worked out.

The specific activities and attributes of successful reflection include a combination of:

- ☐ description;
- ☐ analysis;
- ☐ interpretation;
- ☐ appreciation;
- ☐ self-awareness;
- ☐ self-criticism (what ought to be the case but isn't);
- ☐ imagination (seeing the world through the eyes of others and from as many points of view as possible);
- ☐ creativity (in capturing the richness of the moment in vivid ways);
- ☐ synthesis (making connections between action and theory and general principles - where 'theory' means what others have understood, distilled, made public, and refined against critique).

We look in detail at the characteristics of successful written reflection later in the chapter.

Some historical perspectives

It will already be apparent that systematic and rigorous reflection on professional practice has a considerable history. This section looks briefly at the key educational thinkers associated with it, showing how their ideas have developed, and also offers a glimpse into the history of some professions, showing how reflective practice has established itself as a valuable process in practice development (albeit one which itself is properly open to critical scrutiny and comes with costs as well as benefits). It is not offered in the expectation that readers will pursue these authors, but rather that they recognize the width and depth of serious writing about reflection, and its provenance.

Key historical thinkers in the development of reflection as a serious practice

The notion of learning through experience goes back to the Greeks, where, as we have seen, Aristotle's notions of *praxis* shaped it. *Praxis* is action directed towards the achievement not of an artifact (a thing), but of a virtue (a good in society). It is a form of doing; it is morally informed, morally committed action. Its ends are progressively revised as the 'goods' intrinsic to practice endlessly develop, and are thus determinable in principle, but, as Carr points out:

'What they are at any given time can only be made intelligible in terms of the inherited and largely unarticulated body of practical knowledge which constitutes the traditions within which the good intrinsic to that practice is enshrined. To practise is never a matter of individuals accepting and implementing some rational account of what the aims of their practice should be. It is always a matter of being initiated into the knowledge, understandings and beliefs bequeathed by that tradition through which the practice has been conveyed to us in its present shape.'

(Carr, 1995, p. 68)

To practise is to 'act within a tradition', but also to critique it and contribute to its evolution. It is the very continuing presence of contesting philosophical viewpoints that provides the oppositional tension, which is essential for critical thinking to perform this role.

That is why the development of reflective approaches to learning to be a surgeon is currently vital. It is one means of preventing the profession from being reduced to accepting as unopposed, a list of elements of practice and an account of what to do and how to do it in surgery, constructed by those largely outside the profession, and purporting to have resolved all tensions about what characterizes surgical work.

The ideas of Aristotle have more recently been rehearsed for us by Carr and Grundy (as will be clear from our references to them), and elaborated in the work particularly of Boud, Keogh and Walker; Dewey; Habermas; Kolb; Schön; and Van Manen. The following offers the briefest of glimpses of their contributions. All of them are within the broad tradition that holds it important that people become personally engaged in the learning process and that this involves: experience; observation and reflection; abstract reconceptualisation; and experimentation.

The work of Dewey (1859-1952) and Habermas (whose main relevant writings appeared in the early 1970s) has been described as 'the backbone of the study of reflection' (Moon, 1999, p. 11). It is interesting to note that the ideas fundamental to reflective practice come to us both from America and Europe (John Dewey being an American psychologist, philosopher and educator, and Jurgen Habermas being a German philosopher). They were both interested in how reflection generates knowledge, but they described reflection in different ways and were interested in it for different reasons. Dewey's work focused on the processes of reflection, and sees its motivation as coming from perplexity about practice, in order to make sense of the world. For him, reflection was an active, persistent and careful consideration of belief and knowledge. His writing on reflection uses metaphors of creation, construction, or reconstruction of new identities and meanings, rather than mirror metaphors of re-presentation, image formation, or copying what already exists. He emphasized the link between thought (as reflection) and action in the development of practice. His key educational books include: *My Pedagogic Creed* (1897); *How We Think* (1910; revised ed., 1933); and *Democracy and Education* (1916), of which the second listed is most centrally on reflection. For Habermas, reflection was a tool to be used in developing particular forms of knowledge. His work drives towards the ideals of empowerment and emancipation (see Chapter 3). For him, reflection is about critique, evaluation and liberation. His key work in this field is to be found in his: *Towards a Rational Society* (1971); *Knowledge and Human Interests* (1972); and *Theory and Practice* (1974). He sees knowledge not as out there waiting to be found but as something which people construct together.

Dewey's work gave rise to Kolb's ideas about a 'reflective cycle' (an early model of reflection), which is a rather simplistic view that reflection is generated by experience and feeds back into developed practice and further evaluation. The key points on his cycle were: concrete experience; reflective observation; abstract conceptualization; and active experimentation (Kolb, 1984). Kolb's work was specifically within the field of experiential education (where the focus is on learning through activities), and was taken up within the education of professionals, where a practice was being learnt or developed. This was extended by Gibbs in 1988, to include the following points in a continuous cycle or spiral: description (what happened?); feelings; evaluation (what was good or bad about the experience?); analysis; conclusion (what else would you have done?); and action plan (if it arose again, what would you do?). This rather implies that it is possible to apply directly and quickly to practice that which has been learnt through reflection, which in turn suggests an applicatory relationship between theory and practice. (This idea we, as authors, reject.)

Other work which was founded in Dewey's, and which cannot be ignored even in the briefest summary, is that of Van Manen, and Boud, Keogh and Walker, (1985). Van Manen (whose work has mainly appeared between the 1970s and the 1990s), offers a reflective model of a different shape (hierarchical rather than circular), and contributes the notion of levels of reflection: the first level being about practical concerns in terms of what works; the second being concerned with evaluation of action and belief (practice and theory) and the debating of principles and goals; the third being concerned with ethical and political concerns (the link between practice and broader social issues); and (later) the fourth being concerned with meta-level understanding (higher level ideas about thinking itself). (See Van Manen, 1977.) He also characterized reflection as mindfulness or attentiveness (Van Manen, 1991). The idea of mindfulness highlights the all-pervasive requirement that professionals regard their judgements as provisional and qualified by conditions of uncertainty of both facts and values. This critical, mindful quality of reflection implies a holistic outlook. Here, practitioners maintain ongoing critical questioning of all dimensions of their practice in the light of prevailing professional aims and social values.

Some of this thinking about reflection does not specifically link it to learning, but in the work of Boud, Keogh and Walker, (1985), we have a modern example of *praxis*, in which reflection is specifically seen as turning experience into learning. Their book offers a wide range of examples of ways in which to reflect on professional practice, and indicates the costs in terms and resources, as well as the benefits.

The most influential writer on reflection (and particularly reflection on professional practice) in the last three decades has been Donald Schön, whose key books are: *The Reflective Practitioner* (1983); *Educating the Reflective Practitioner* (1987), which outlined his main thinking; and *The Reflective Turn* (1991), which provided case studies in and on educational practice. He focused on the preparation of professionals and particularly on their learning in, and from, the practice setting, which he characterized as the 'swampy lowlands' because practice happens in the indeterminate zone (of life), and is always by definition, complex and incomplete. He began with a more down-to-earth understanding of the nature of professional practice, and therefore saw the importance of context in considering and learning from practical experience.

Schön's work, though much critiqued, has contributed most to the general drive to incorporate reflection into the teaching of professional practice in professional settings. He teased apart the artistry from the rule-following 'craft or rationality' of practice, which he saw as dangerous. From him we get the idea of reflection-in-action (the thinking that happens when actions do not go according to plan) and reflection-on-action (reflection that occurs after the action), and the need for professionals to learn in a sheltered practicum (an experience of practice where the student has a taste of real practice but does not bear the full responsibility for every aspect of the work). (It is this last idea that we have adapted for surgical education in Chapter 4.) Schön described the main features of a practicum as: 'learning by doing, coaching rather than teaching, and a dialogue of reciprocal reflection-in-action between coach and student' (Schön, 1987, p 303).

Schön's work has been criticized for using imprecise terms (there is debate about what reflection-in-action really means, and his definition seems too narrow), and on the grounds that his practical examples do not exactly match his theorizing. For example, Eraut, (1995), wishes to reject the term 'reflection' as Schön uses it, and Greenwood, (1993), points out inconsistencies (in his work with Argyris) between Schön's ideas and his actual pedagogical interventions as described and recommended in his work. Interestingly, Greenwood recommends that nurse educators should follow Schön's theorizing rather than his practice. Nonetheless, Schön's work was pioneering, and remains seminal for those who educate professionals in the practice setting.

The history of reflective practice in health care

The history of the development of reflection in health care, although it goes back at least 25 years in Britain, America and Australia, has not yet been written. Nonetheless, it is already possible to say that it will need to refer to the work of the following: Benner, (1984); Carper, (1978); Driscoll, (2000); Fish, Twinn and Purr, (1989); Freshwater, (2002); Johns, (2002); and Rolfe, (2000), in nursing; Higgs (who has published a wide range of books in the 1990s and 21st Century) in physiotherapy; and Mattingly and Fleming, (1994), and Ryan (1995), and Ryan *et al*, (2003), in occupational therapy. Many of these authors have also been involved in developing postgraduate work at masters level within their profession, and a number of PhDs from across these professions and based on a reflective methodology are now on the shelves of a number of universities.

By comparison with all these, there is, so far, only a handful of names to report across the entire medical field, and all their work is much more recent. The key figures are: (from America) Epstein's 1999 work on 'mindful practice', which is an excellent summary of how reflective practice relates to medicine; (from Australia) the work of Cox, (1999), in surgery; (from Britain) the work of Downie and Macnaughton, (2000), and Greenhalgh and Hurwitz, (1998), in medicine generally; West, (2001), in general practice; and White and Stancombe (2003), in paediatrics. In addition, it should be recognized that the writing of Gawande, (2001), in surgery (produced in America but published in Britain) is also in the reflective tradition, although he does not make this explicit. Further, there are in England now, several masters courses in education in clinical settings for medical consultants and other senior staff, in which reflective practice is an integral component, and several on-going PhDs in the field of medical education on the artistry of practice and reflection are known to us, and one that has recently been successful.

When the history of reflection in health care is collated and presented, it will need to take account of the increasing work in inter-professional health care teams (which will spread the value of reflection further). In our view this will need to attend to the following, (many of which Rose and Best, (2005) forthcoming, begins to tackle):

- ❏ the different definitions of clinical supervision, clinical education and mentoring in different health care professions;
- ❏ the different activities and philosophies which emerge from these;
- ❏ the early use of (reliance on) models - some of which were designed as frameworks but were taken as rigid requirements;
- ❏ the discovery that it can be a manager's tool and can even backfire on practitioners who write open and honest reflections which they assumed would be honoured as private but which were required as evidence in courts of law (see, for example, Cotton, 2001);
- ❏ a move towards a freeing up of definitions and a turning towards critical enquiry as the central activity.

This is the context for looking more closely at what is most valuable for learning surgeons (and their surgical teachers) to reflect upon, and how this might best be done.

What surgeons might reflect on and how they might do so

As we have already indicated in our overview, for professional practitioners and especially those seeking to develop their practice, reflection mostly begins with an incident from their own practice. It is then possible to focus the reflection itself more widely or narrowly (looking more deeply at the particular practice or using the event as a springboard to consider wider professional, social and political aspects). The discipline of reflective practice is at least partly about looking rigorously at one's own practice, however, and no educational portfolio assembled by learning surgeons would be complete without some attempts at an in-depth study of their own practice, properly illuminated by reference to wider ideas and understanding.

Exploring holistic surgical practice through reflection

Trainers mostly reject the significance of reflection on practice, see as important only the surface features of practice, emphasize the end product of learning, and seek its evidence through assessment. Thus, there is little requirement of the trainee to explore practice, and the major activity in the course of all this, is the assessor's, not the learner's. Here, it is seen as enough that practice is divided into single elements, which are scrutinized by an assessor who will observe each one, and tick them off appropriately. This contributes little to the learner's self-knowledge and ability to self-assess. It is piecemeal, rather than holistic, and often leads to highly artificial assessments in the practice setting, because in reality practice is not piecemeal and no practitioner in the course of a clinical event or activity calls upon only one element of practice. This must mean that much of the important contextualizing detail which will in reality affect the quality of the learner's practice, is excluded in the effort to be 'objective' by narrowing the assessment focus to competencies. See Chapter 6 for more detail about this.

By contrast, we are advocating the recognition that practice is an holistic activity, and deserves to be developed and assessed as such. Crucially, this cannot be wisely developed or justly assessed unless much of what is *not* visible is also taken account of. Further, we would argue that the learner is the person who should be most active, that evidence of a learner's development is best accrued and demonstrated by the learner, and that such documentation will become the best evidence for the learner's achievements (or lack of them).

For learning surgeons, we would argue, it is essential for wise development of practice and just assessment of it, that learners provide evidence of all that underlies and drives their practice. For this purpose, reflection is the best process. It enables the learner to focus on a complete event, activity or experience within their own practice, and to unearth much that lies under it. (Since there is an element of mystery at the core of all professional practice, we do not argue for an attempt to be exhaustive about this.)

We believe that the following elements of practice should be brought together in an account of practice, and that they should be clarified and refined by talking it through and/or writing it up.

In order to acknowledge the holistic character of a piece of practice, the following should be focused on.

1. **The context of that individual and particular practice event/action**
    This means noting carefully the features of and influences upon the particular event/action/activity which has been chosen for detailed exploration, and the factors which shaped what the practitioner brought to the event on that occasion.

2. **The professional dimensions of professional practice**
    This means considering those aspects of practice that are driven by or are affected by our values and stance as members of a profession (see Chapter 2).

3. **The personal dimensions of professional practice**
    This means being alert to how our personal professional beliefs, assumptions, theories and values impact on our conduct in practice and how our practice has impacted upon them (see page 27).

4. **The clinical thinking that is used during action**
    This involves being able to explain, share and critique (most of) the thinking processes we call upon in practice (see Chapters 7 and 8).

5. **The knowing that is drawn on during action**
    This involves being able to identify, explore and critique (most of) the knowledge we draw upon in practice (see Chapter 9).

6. **How this relates to wider views of practice**
    This involves being able to relate all this to the wider traditions of practice in this profession and to critique both those traditions and our practice.

We offer below comments on ways of exploring this, and provide an overview of assessment in Chapter 6. In Part two, we expand in detail and provide examples of simple and speedy ways of writing up this sort of reflection, and how it can be used for assessment purposes.

Some key processes for reflecting on practice

The minimum requirements for engaging in reflection are:

❑   a mindset in the learner and teacher that seeks to home-in upon those clinical events and actions which (under rigorous reflection) will yield rich understanding;

❑   the willingness to prioritize this process so that time for talking through the full reflection on an event between teacher and learner is provided; and

❐   the motivation (which comes with trying it out) to spend some time writing further about it.

It is arguable, for example, that time between cases could be used for some of this talking (properly prompted by rigorous questions like those offered below), and that protected teaching time could routinely be given to group reflection on a clinical experience. We suggest also that time should be found, both inside and outside the clinical setting, for writing, since it provides learners with perspectives they would not otherwise access. We demonstrate in Part two how written reflection can be built up quickly.

The main processes that will develop good reflective practice are: following a rigorous process for reflection; engaging in dialogue with teachers or peers; and recognizing the proper ethical and moral obligations to patients and colleagues. We offer some comments on each, and then follow these by: providing some useful starting points for reflection; showing how critical incidents can be used; and providing some guidelines for exploring an event in surgical practice. At the end of this section we also provide references to support those wishing to explore the autobiographical and the narrative approaches.

Following a rigorous process for reflection

We offer some guidelines for this, but eventually each reflection will grow into a structure that is right for a given individual who is describing and exploring an event which is particular to them. This is because reflection needs to be exploratory and to pursue what arises rather than provide answers to protocol questions.

Engaging in dialogue with teachers or peers

This dialogue can occur in both talking and writing with anyone who shared the event being reflected on, and particularly the following:

❐   teachers (which might include anyone in the entire surgical team: nurses, and Operating Department Practitioners (ODPs) for example are already well practised in reflection);
❐   peers, which might include senior learners from other professions (nurses learning to be First Assistants in theatre or assistant surgical practitioners, anaesthetists learning in theatre, or nurses learning in theatre, on wards or in clinics).

Recognizing the proper ethical and moral obligations to patients and colleagues

Clearly a professional discussion of a case is a natural part of learning in surgery, and where the environment in which it takes place is professional and confidential, the patient's name and details will be used. However, wherever these details are recorded in writing for the purpose of reflection, proper codes of conduct must be put in place to protect the patient's and even colleagues' identity. Names, places and times must be changed, and it is often useful to turn two or three cases into one, taking the salient features from each. This is important even if the only reader is expected to be the writer, and is vital if the writing is to be shared (which we would encourage). This is by no means as difficult as it sounds. Indeed, we have done just that in the examples offered in Part two, but they demonstrably still provide real and serious examples of important learning opportunities.

All this points up and emphasizes the comments we made in Chapter 4 about the importance of professional conversation between teacher and learner. This is certainly the key means of developing reflection. It can take the form of one-to-one discussion between teacher and learner, or between learner and learner, and can be of particular use within a group where that group is the entire theatre team (see Chapter 10).

Starting points for reflection

The clinical setting is so rich in experiences that are worth reflecting on, that most learners will need little help in starting. However, we offer the following as useful additional starting points. In all the following, writers should try to find appropriate ways of illuminating practice with theory and vice-versa.

Suitable starting points for reflection are as follows.

- ❏ Talk to a colleague and make notes as you go (or use a dictaphone).
- ❏ Describe in detail a moment of practice which has surprised you or provided you with a sudden insight.
- ❏ Write a letter to a friend.
- ❏ Write an e-mail to a friend or colleague.
- ❏ Use questions about a piece of practice offered by others (see below).
- ❏ Generate your own questions.
- ❏ Make a list of key points and expand them.
- ❏ Create diagrams and concept-maps of the practice and related issues.
- ❏ Write freely in a brainstorm session.
- ❏ Take a sentence from something you have read or heard that has sparked your interest.
- ❏ Start your thinking with an image (metaphor/simile) or an object that is important to you as a symbol of how an event has seemed.
- ❏ Remember that you can reflect further on a piece of writing you have already done.
- ❏ Share your writing with a colleague and take up an issue which emerges.
- ❏ Reflect on the act - and the kind of product - of writing itself (and how it compared with talk).
- ❏ Write about yourself as a learner (in a range of different settings).
- ❏ Experiment with a variety of forms (prose, poetry, drama, drawing, maps, diagrams)
- ❏ Finding your own voice in writing is important (see below).

These ideas have been influenced by the work of Jennifer Moon, (1999), pp. 120-133.

Using critical incidents

A critical incident in reflection is not the same as an adverse incident in medicine. In education, a critical incident is an event whose significance has been produced by the way we look at it. The incident, which can be a very ordinary happening, is imbued with importance by the practitioner for whom the incident raises a question or poses a value conflict.

Using critical incidents rests on the understanding that learning is a response to both experience and personal interest. In order to move beyond our everyday, working way of looking at things we need to arrest experience in a way that renders it open to analysis and critique.

The ways in which critical incidents can be exploited in order to learn from them include:

- ❏ journal keeping or recording field notes;
- ❏ extended writing;
- ❏ critical friendship, critical companionship or clinical supervision;
- ❏ group reflection and discussion;
- ❏ e-mail discussion.

An example of guidelines developed specifically for surgeons

The following shown in Table 5.1 offers one way of examining an event of surgical practice in order to look in detail at the elements that we recommended learners to focus on (see page 73).

The work of David Tripp (1993) and Boud, Keogh and Walker, (1985), provide many examples of reflection which has started with an autobiographical critical incident. For help with building up a series of autobiographical pieces into a large whole, see the work of Winter, *et al*, (1999), and for work on narrative in medicine, see Greenhalgh and Hurwitz, (1998).

Writing reflectively: some starting points

Reflective writing has the potential to make the knowledge embedded in our practice more explicit and accessible and more open to development.

We have already indicated the need for writing reflectively in surgery. This section therefore identifies the key advantages of so doing; offers some indications of what characterizes successful reflective writing, and makes some brief comments on how to develop and refine such writing.

Table 5:1 Surgical strands of reflection - a prompt sheet. Main questions in bold, prompts bulleted (adapted from: Fish and Twinn, 1997).

A. THE FACTUAL STRAND:
Give a descriptive narrative of the event (what happened, and what you felt, thought and did about it)
- Describe the context of the practical situation.
- What happened, how did you think, feel and act, and why?
- What were the key moments of the event?
- How do you see these? (Consider them critically)?

B. THE RETROSPECTIVE STRAND
Look at the event as a whole. What patterns and possible new meanings can you see? (But this is still about surface performance)
- What are the main patterns of: (for example: reason and/or motive, activities, failures, successes, emotions, frustrations, limitations, constraints, coercions)?
- How might others (patients/fellow team members/observers) have seen it overall?
- Analyse the oral language used between self and fellow professionals.

C. THE SUB-STRATUM STRAND
What assumptions, beliefs, values, reasoning and judgements underlay the events?
- What have you learnt about being a member of a profession?
- What beliefs, assumptions, theories, and values, shaped your conduct?
- What customs, traditions, rituals, beliefs, dogmas, prejudices, were brought to/endemic in the situation? Where did they come from?
- What knowledge was used or created during the event?
- What beliefs are emerging about knowledge and how it is gained/used/created ?
- What perspectives from formal theory and personal experience and theory shaped the event?
- What does the event (and these reflections) tell us about how you view theory and practice?
- What key thinking processes did you engage in?
- What key professional judgements were made during practice?
- What moral and ethical issues were raised for you by this experience?
- How do you regard these now?

D. THE CONNECTIVE STRAND
Relate what you have learnt in the above strands to the wider world - of practice ideas, reflections, theories and actions of other professionals, and (via reading) to formal theory
- How does it relate to past experiences, and how will it relate to future ones?
- What issues and practices in your own work will you now explore further?
- What theories might you develop for/about future action?
- What do you need to find out more about? How will you do this?
- What explorations/investigations of future practice might you plan?

The key differences between talking and writing reflectively

The following table offers a summary of some key differences between spoken and written reflection.

Table 5:2 Talking and writing reflectively.

Talking reflectively:	Writing reflectively:
• can be used to explore ideas and make them one's own (can be dialogic)	• often reveals more than one sets out to say and teaches one what one thinks (can be dialogic)
• can happen in the action	• rarely occurs during action
• is time limited by events and ephemeral	• is enduring and often leads to special satisfaction
• is rough and ready	• can be reshaped
• is personal and seems subjective	• is personal but can seem more objective
• is quick to produce and to hear	• takes longer to write and to read
• is unlikely to be perfectly ordered and clear	• can be given shape and balance
• cannot stop and look back over points made and so cannot easily refine them	• can review points at all stages and so can refine them
• is no good for exploring intricate ideas and complex arguments	• can present arguments and connections more clearly
• is no good for comparing complex facts and figures	• can make comparisons easily
• means it is hard to hold enough in the head to keep all ideas coherent	• can work on coherence at all points
• is face to face and very direct	• enables you to express some things you could not easily say
• means ideas are fragile. Interruptions can cause loss of thought and progress can be blocked	• is more robust. You can come back later, and add to it or refine or change it
• means you can discover what you have to say as you go, but you have to be quick and can't unsay something once it has been said	• allows more time to discover what you want to say and how best to say it
• can be artistic in content and form but only if rehearsed	• can be artistic in content and form and extends the power to find the right words
• can be inhibited by the social context	• enables you to adopt an unusual or private role

The key characteristics of reflective writing

The following characteristics of reflective writing are offered as a guide to those beginning. Further guidance is given in Part two in respect of specific elements of practice which the learning surgeon may find it helpful to write about.

Reflective writing:

- is about concrete situations;
- uses the first person singular - is autobiographical;
- seeks to understand an action/event which has been personally experienced;
- is 'in the moment';
- attends in detail to the context of the action/event being reflected on;
- seeks to study an event/action more deeply and to unpack the thinking and knowing beneath its surface, as well as the values, beliefs, assumptions, and theories that drove the writer's actions;
- describes wholes rather than parts;
- is narrative in style;
- shows evidence of learning (deepening understanding);
- sometimes uses figurative language (rich descriptions based on, for example, comparisons as in similes and metaphors);
- demonstrates commitment to professional ideals and uses these as a touchstone to critique practice;
- takes account of the views and perspectives of others involved in the action or event;
- identifies factors contributing to the situation which may be historical, political, economic, social, ethical, autobiographical, and psychological;
- draws attention to what may previously have been taken for granted, rendering the familiar strange;
- enriches experience by the acquisition of new perspectives;
- seeks relationships to wider theory and general principles.

Some suggestions for refining reflective writing

The relationship between writer, subject and audience is what shapes writing. The writer can use the following to shape the reader's response. (They are not separate matters but are delicately interrelated.)

- Form (this is the overall structure of the piece of writing, which can be given shape towards the end, or, preferably naturally begins to shape itself as one works on it).
- Style (the sentence shape, the repetition, the figures of speech).
- Tone (the writer's attitude to subject/content, which would emerge if it were read aloud).
- Voice (the personal sound and style of the writer which come from an amalgam of all the above).

It is also important before you begin to think about your intentions for self and audience, to present your credentials as a writer on your subject, and to have an idea of the audience you are writing for (you need to sense them looking over your shoulder). By means of working over a piece of reflective writing, it is possible to adjust it in whatever way helps to emphasize the above factors. Reading the work through *aloud* will help writers hear what else needs to be done to it (correct typos and enhance further the good parts).

Voice is very important in writing. Successful writing depends greatly on creating a voice which is appropriate to the writer, the subject and the intentions of the work. Voice is the means of carrying content. Writers need to enable their audience to place the voice of their writing, and readers need to be able to recognize, through hearing the voice, the writer's emotions about and attitude to self, subject, and audience. It is tone of voice which tells the audience how to interpret what is being conveyed - whether it is intended to be comic, satiric, sad, thoughtful - and which thus gives the audience a starting point from which to respond. Voice is created through vocabulary, subject reference points, use of tense and person of verb, precision of syntax, repetition, use of figurative language, tone, emphasis, transcribed pronunciation. It conveys much about the writer beyond what the writer is saying - or, put another way, it offers a further context in which to place and through which to understand what is conveyed in words. It can convey highly significant matters like age, gender, experience of life and topic (see Fish, 1998, p. 230).

In seeking to extend and enrich writing, it is useful to think of the reader as a specific person who knows relatively little about the detail of one's practice but who is really interested in trying to understand it and how you see it. Ask yourself what such a reader needs to know.

It is also important to keep clarifying the purpose of one's writing. Considering the following might help.

- ❐ Tell it (your incident/experience/insight) as it seemed. Don't fudge it, don't hedge, but expect your understanding of it to change as you work over it more.
- ❐ Look for places where you have assumed that the reader knows details they don't really. Make these far more explicit.
- ❐ Say far more about the context (your beliefs, values, theories, your views about professional practice, what is relevant about your own personal history).
- ❐ Say something about the moral and/or ethical dimensions of your incident.
- ❐ Think carefully about the structure of your writing. Have you used all necessary conventions available to the writer to control how the reader meets your work? (e.g. title, sections, headings, sub-headings, lists). Remember, headings may change as the writing develops.
- ❐ Think carefully about the order in which you tell the reader about things. Would a different order enable you better to highlight certain issues or make the reader better able to share your reactions to events?
- ❐ Add some more rich texture to your writing. Describe more vividly what it was like to be there. Find similes to help the reader sense what it was really like to be there. Find metaphors to give impact to your descriptions.

❑   Think about your written style. It needs to be autobiographical, but even then there is a huge range of tone of voice available to you.

❑   The shape and sound of sentences is what gives character to writing. Look at yours as if you were reading it for the first time. What needs clarifying?

❑   Think about the relationship you want to have with your audience. Different purposes for writing demand of the writer different forms of credibility. What is appropriate in the particular context?

❑   Think carefully about what the reader needs to know about you as writer in order to relate to what is written and to know how to respond to it.

❑   A small piece of autobiographical writing which is designed mainly to explore ideas and the development of values and understanding may well stand alone, without reference to other information, other writers and other ideas.

❑   But if the writing is intended to explore practice critically, and share this with others who have an interest in the same area, then it is necessary to connect this piece of writing to the ideas of the outside world.

❑   This means turning to the literature on the subject, whose role is to enrich the thinking, the exploring, the complexity of ideas, and to link the writing to its place in the world of those ideas.

For further information about accentuating themes, highlighting contrasts, using fresher language (removing clichés), and simplifying writing, see Fish, (1998), pp. 232/3.

End note

Equipped with an understanding in principle about reflection and its role in learning, we shall now turn to the role of assessment in teaching and learning. In Part two, we provide concrete examples of reflective writing and at the end of Part two we indicate ways forward in investigating educational practice by using reflection as one means of educational research.

Chapter 6

Assessment and its role in education for clinical practice: an overview

---

Introduction
    The intentions of this chapter
    The historical context

An overview of assessment and its role in teaching and learning
    Definition of assessment
    The nature of assessment
    Assessment within three different models of the curriculum
    The vital distinction between competence and competencies

What should be assessed in surgical practice and by what means?
    What should be assessed in the clinical setting to educate thinking surgeons?
    The principles that should guide that assessment
    What are the key elements of assessment for surgeons?

Introduction

At a time of changing demands and expectations in surgical practice, it is essential for surgical teachers to understand and engage in new levels of debate about, and new practices in, assessment and its role in the clinical setting. The unacceptable alternative is for surgeons to become the passive recipients of educational decisions made for them by those who do not know surgery from the inside. The educational problem is clear. Assessment should play a central role in learning in all contexts. Yet currently, learners emerge from a surgical attachment with only the most general of evidence of their progress, no clear indication of their specific abilities in clinical processes or technical and operative procedures, and no record of how they conduct themselves in the clinical setting both as surgeons and as learners. It is inconceivable that this state of affairs will be allowed to continue long into the 21st Century.

The intentions of this chapter

Accordingly, we seek to equip readers to begin to develop more appropriate ways of assessing learning surgeons in the current changing clinical environment, and specifically within the clinical setting. The development of clinical assessment must be underpinned by sound foundations, which must include an informed educational understanding. Such understanding must relate to: the key questions which assessment raises for educators; the thrust of the educational arguments and main schools of educational thinking which can shape responses to those questions; and the appropriate and accurate language in which to debate, choose and plan assessment, and which is also shared by all other educators throughout health care.

The key questions are: What is the nature of assessment? What role should it play within education, and particularly in education in clinical settings? How can it be used to chart progress in clinical practice? What should be assessed within the clinical setting and by whom; and how can a robust gate-keeping process be established?

This chapter therefore offers in its first main section an overview of assessment generally, and contains a broad definition of it. It also reveals how different conceptions of the nature of assessment arise, and illustrates a range of schools of thought about teaching and learning, and competence and competencies. Each one of these ways of thinking shapes a crucially different role for assessment, some of which are more appropriate than others for use in the clinical setting. In a second section, it then focuses on the assessment of surgeons within the clinical setting, showing what should be assessed in order to create reliable evidence of their overall educational and clinical achievements, and how this can be done in a robust, disciplined, valid and reliable way, which leads into a sound gate-keeping process at the end of the attachment or the programme. It considers the vital role in all this of the surgeon educator's professional judgement. In offering these things, we also seek to debunk some of the current myths that bedevil clear thinking about these matters in relation to cultivating a thinking surgeon.

The historical context

The wider context of medicine generally is well set by Coles, who reminds us that: 'For much of the past one hundred years, the assessment of doctors has relentlessly pursued an 'objective' (and hence psychometric) approach', attempting to measure what doctors do and 'match these measurements against agreed and observable criteria for doctors' behaviour'. As Coles points out, this attempt has failed, so that, 'rather than pursuing the increasingly discredited 'psychometric' approach to objective assessment, our future must lie in understanding and developing (rather than ignoring or dismissing) the subjective judgments we make' (Coles, 2000).

It is important within this context, to understand the present situation in respect of surgical assessment, and how it has emerged. History answers the questions: Where are we? Why are we where we are? This sub-section considers these in respect of the role of assessment in the clinical setting, and seeks to show why surgeons (who are experts in their profession of surgery and traditionally have been, and will remain, the key teachers in the development of this discipline), have only recently recognized the imperative need to attend to assessment in the practice setting.

In the past, particularly in the last two decades of the 20th Century, the long time spent in years of training by surgical registrars as the key apprentices to expert surgeons, resulted in their developing a repertoire of frequently practised clinical processes and procedures. They thus almost inevitably became well-experienced consultant surgeons, who had been ratified by their masters, as ready for a career in, and able to give sound support to, the NHS. The Royal College formal examinations largely tested their theoretical knowledge but the knowledge of their ability to manage a ward, run a clinic and undertake increasingly complex operations was passed between consultants and other persons involved in their promotion, on an informal, word of mouth basis. This ratification of their achievements within their clinical working environment was the *only* means of assessing their clinical practice. But it was a mere formality, and technically did not merit the term 'assessment'. That is, it neither drew upon, nor generated, robust detailed documentation of specific achievements within clinical practice, nor were the decisions and judgements made of the learner by the teacher either transparent or based upon clearly defined criteria.

Today, however, there no longer exists plentiful time and opportunity for learning surgical practice, and surgeons are less experienced at all stages of their careers than in the past. Thus, on two counts more must be gained (in both depth and breadth) from each of the fewer experiences available to learning surgeons. As a result, the capabilities that are built by them need to be carefully documented for use by those who plan the service, as well as by subsequent teachers. Further, accountability now demands that all professionals collect robust and detailed evidence of their achievement at all stages. This is now recognized everywhere as vital, in order to ensure patient safety, to equip learners properly for their future careers, and to protect the teacher in the face of possible litigation should patients come to harm or other things go wrong with that career.

All this has arisen because of recent changes in specialty practice, in the law, and in society's ideas both about accountability and about the relationship of leisure time and work time. These have seriously destabilized the previous conditions for learning, and demand new approaches. New pressures exist too because society's trust in professionals (both clinicians and teachers) has also been eroded by incidents like those at Bristol and Alder Hey, which have highlighted the lack of rigorous self-regulation by the profession, and have resulted in significant new government regulation. The current pressures for multi-professional team working are also bringing changes. Until recently, old traditions of how to produce a surgeon and of what matters in learning to be a surgeon, tended to isolate surgery from other health care professions whose educational understanding has been developed and extended in the last two decades. This has contributed to the surgical profession's slowness to recognize that education as a whole is as vital to a profession's development as is its scientific research base.

This is not to deny that there has been some recognition of the significance of assessment within the surgical profession. It is true that there has been what is referred to as an annual assessment of surgeons in training, since the 1970s. It began with senior registrars (then the only formally recognized training post) with a formal but unstructured annual review process. With the reorganisation of higher surgical training by Kenneth Calman in the 1990s and the rationalisation of senior registrar and registrar posts into the new Specialist Registrar category, it became mandatory annually for doctors to have their Record of In-service Training, Assessed (to be 'RITA-ed'). It will be noted, though, that this apparently summative assessment process, for which the postgraduate deans are held responsible, is not a direct assessment of doctors in the clinical setting, but rather an assessment of their record over the year (not itself the product of a rigorous assessment process, but rather of a sign off procedure which is sometimes carried out by seniors without a face-to-face discussion with the learner involved)! Assessment here has not been conceived of as a central activity of a rigorous process of teaching and learning, but rather as an isolated one-off activity, and neither has it been supported by educational input for the key teachers involved. It is therefore hardly surprising that the RITA process is little respected by consultants, that Surgical Specialist Registrars question its appropriateness and quality, and that there is much variation in the process throughout the UK. Educators too, see little in it that they recognize as educational assessment. That is: it is not based on a serious educational foundation of a logically constructed curriculum (educational programme) in which is embedded an assessment process with a clear educational role; it is not operated in the light of publicly shared criteria, but rather on a sign off procedure where signatures are accrued across the year (but do not give detailed evidence of what the learner has achieved); and it has no educational value, providing no educational challenge to good candidates and occurring too late in the programme to benefit weaker candidates. Thus, although it is supposed to be a gate-keeping process, its documentation and procedures are not robust enough to fail the unsuccessful. The pressure, therefore, is to pass everyone.

The surgical Royal Colleges have over the last ten years responded to these obvious deficits by widening their examinations. Indeed, this decade has seen, as never before, formal examinations in surgery raised to the point of being the main discriminator of surgical prowess and reason for progression. There is some element of practical in these examinations (both simulated and real practice outside the examinee's own clinical setting), but it is surely bizarre that something as practically focused as surgery is not assessed in the examinee's own working practice setting, and that young surgeons' progress through their attachments does not currently draw upon detailed formative practical assessments which give rise to the final record of achievement.

It seems probable that the assessment of surgeons' clinical achievements has been sidelined because of a perception that such assessment involves a subjective process, which is open to bias and abuse, and which cannot be made valid and reliable without an enormous training programme to make surgeon educators competent to assess the very practice they have been teaching and assessing informally for years! In fact, these ideas arise from a total failure to understand the nature of educational assessment and the proper role in it of the professional judgement of consultant teachers (see also Coles, 2000).

All this is no longer merely bizarre. It has gained a much greater seriousness with the new working conditions for surgeons. Now, without sound evidence that good educational processes (of which assessment is a key element) have been attended to with rigour and discipline in the clinical setting, the quality of the surgeon and his/her progress will be in question, and the safety of patients will be seen as at serious risk.

An overview of assessment and its role in teaching and learning

All concepts within education are problematic. That is, there is not, and there never can be, one clearly and universally agreed way of defining, conceiving and utilizing educational ideas and activities. As we have seen in previous chapters, they are values based. That is, one's own personal, professional and educational values dictate how one sees, uses, prioritizes and weighs educational ideas and activities. This means that it is only possible to offer a broad definition of teaching, learning and assessment, and that it is vital to recognize and consider the range of possible ways of conceptualizing and utilizing them, so that informed, logical and intelligent choices can be made, and rationally defended in the light of one's clarified values, intentions and priorities.

These matters, too, are dynamic. Ideas about education and about professional priorities change and develop. Teaching, learning and assessment are activities or practices that evolve as a result of being used and discussed. In health care professions, educational choices must also be made in response to the evolving needs of that profession and its patients, society and the government. Thus, educational programmes should - even must - be eternally developing, and the basis of a given curriculum can therefore only be a temporary agreement. This means that there will be and there needs to be proper and healthy on-going contention within a profession about the nature of practice generally, the nature of the practice of that profession, the nature of the knowledge which underpins it, and how practice currently does, or shortly should, relate to these choices.

This debate is already well attended to in all educationally mature health care professions, and now needs to be begun and sustained in surgery. This means eschewing the current unquestioned assumption that in surgery, educational matters can be 'got right' and cast in tablets of stone. It means abandoning the consequent futile search for the correct curriculum which will contain perfected assessment procedures. It also means that the current worrying refusal to put any assessment in place in the clinical setting until this perfection has been reached, cannot continue.

What we offer here, therefore, is fuel to enable colleagues to engage in an informed way in these debates. Clearly, our own presentation as writers is itself influenced by our own educational and professional values (which we have already indicated in earlier chapters). Readers will therefore need to take this into account as they critique the following and seek to build their own personal educational philosophy.

Definition of assessment

Assessment is an all-embracing term for an educational process that recognizes and records the development and progress of the learner's achievements and/or gives evidence for progression within an educational programme and a career. It covers any of the situations in which an aspect of a learner's education or training is in some sense rigorously measured or otherwise recognized or appreciated, whether this is by a teacher, an examiner, a colleague (peer), or a learner him/herself. This definition is probably broad enough to be agreed by most educators.

We believe that assessment is a fundamental and central activity of teaching and learning (and should never be considered in isolation from it), and that it should always serve an educational purpose or purposes. We note that in practice, measurement (the according of numbers in an assessment process) has not proved an essential element of assessment, neither does it render assessment any more scientific and objective than is assessment which uses written comments. Indeed, where there is need to communicate between teachers with rigour and discipline about a learner's abilities, written comment is often less open than are numbers to ambiguity about the learner's actual achievements. Assessment is also often seen as specifically related to tests and examinations, but neither is essential to it. Indeed, the value of any assessment is ultimately governed by whether it was worth doing in the first place (by its educational value). This means that assessment for its own sake without a proper educational purpose, is valueless, and some kinds of examinations and over-assessment within university courses (where the learner is subject to an unreasonable number of assessments in too short a period), are commonly seen as examples of this.

Broadly speaking then, educational assessment is concerned with demonstrating how well, and in what ways, a learner has profited from the learning opportunities provided, and with recording these achievements and the learner's educational progress. Assessment must also play a key role in the gate-keeping process for entry to various levels of a profession.

However much it can be dressed up in percentages, graphs, curves of distribution or plain numbers, assessment is no more an exact science than is medicine. Decisions by assessors about what numbers to accord to a learner's achievement are themselves interpretations and do not represent absolute facts. Assessment thus inevitably involves some subjectivity, and we believe that there is not and never will be, a method that will overcome this. Indeed, the assessment by a teacher of a learner's achievements is very like the diagnostic processes used in medicine. Evidence and logic naturally contribute to a teacher's and a doctor's conclusions about learner or patient, but professional judgement will inevitably be a key component.

In fact, teachers make judgements about learners all the time. These are an *informal* form of assessment. In this respect, teachers are like doctors. They find themselves, as part of their ingrained thinking processes, making everyday, on-going judgements and coming to informal conclusions (see also Table 4:1, p. 55). Such assessments (which sometimes are based on unfounded and unsubstantiated assumptions) are often crucial for the learner, for teachers, as well as for institutions, the profession and the public. Teachers therefore, need to be vigilant about how and why they make them. Indeed, in order to be fair, such judgements must be part of a well-planned process, use public criteria, and involve multiple perspectives (more than one view), and they must be principled. Further, learners and all those who receive the results must be aware of what principles are at work. It should also be noted that a coherent system of assessment crystallizes for learners and the public/society the priorities and values of those who set it up, and who, as a result inevitably promote a particular set of educational and professional values.

Assessment is often undertaken because we are interested in 'outcomes' and 'standards'. The public expects a profession to have standards set in respect of the special responsibilities associated with professional practice. All members of that profession are expected to understand and meet these standards. Those entering the profession need to understand their responsibility with respect to these standards, but it should be remembered that standards are themselves a notional and arbitrary hurdle, and that outcomes cannot be fully understood in isolation from the learner and the particular situation and context in which they were reached. Underpinning any standards (whether this is recognized or not) there will be a set of values with moral and ethical dimensions which are related to the profession's view of what constitutes good practice. It is wise for a profession to make these explicit and examine them carefully to be sure that they genuinely represent their key espoused values, since learners and others who are exposed to them will construe them as such.

The nature of assessment

The nature of assessment for professional education (like that of teaching and learning within which assessment should sit) should be determined by the nature of the professional practice in which the learner is engaging (what it is really like 'as it is lived'), and the nature of the knowledge base that underpins that professional practice (see also Coles, 2000). These, of course, are open to interpretation. How they are conceived will depend upon one's values and world view, and will determine the kinds of education offered to learners, and the kind of learner to be produced. There is thus a proper educational logic to these matters and we flout, ignore or are ignorant of it, at our peril (see Fish and Coles, 2005).

This is a deeply serious matter. If attention is not carefully paid to this primary analysis of the nature of the professional practice being learnt and assessed, and the nature of its knowledge base, then the only alternative is to pick methods of assessment pragmatically out of the air or out of someone else's educational programme, whose logic will never exactly fit our own situation. Then, there will be a major distortion not only of the assessment process (which will provide inaccurate, inappropriate or even irrelevant results), but also the teaching and learning that surrounds it will be misdirected and the professional who emerges from this will not be what they appear to be on paper. This is why a curriculum (a whole, logically connected overview of an educational programme: its intentions; educational activities like teaching, learning and assessment; its content, and its philosophy), has to be built carefully from proper foundations. It is why a central tenet of good curriculum design is that it is inappropriate to impose on any profession a whole curriculum from another country, culture or profession, because the nature of professional practice and the knowledge underpinning it are context specific and individual to a culture and its values.

Even within a given culture there are choices to be made. Some British surgeons, for example, will see the nature of clinical practice as mainly technical (about acquiring surgical and medical skills, and scientific knowledge which can be applied to that practice). This would mean surgeons acquiring knowledge in order to apply it, and gaining training in skills that they can reproduce accurately, on all occasions. This would produce a surgeon who saw him/herself primarily as a technician. Here, the assessment will be about assessing the knowledge by examination and the skills in a neutral environment from which all other confounding factors have been excluded. Success here will be interpreted as the efficient and accurate reproduction of both the knowledge and the skills. The means of recording this would be the kind of ticked boxes associated with competency-based assessment (which we discuss below).

We would argue, that such a view of assessment overlooks a number of highly significant matters, as follows.

- ❐   It ignores the thinking that lies behind the skills.
- ❐   It does not focus on how, in real practice, surgeons adapt their knowledge and improvise their skill.
- ❐   It does not require them to be aware of and confront their own attitudes, values, assumptions, beliefs and personal theories which are part of the context of their practice and which drive their actions.
- ❐   It does not make central the moral and ethical dimensions of their patients' needs.
- ❐   It does not focus on how rounded a professional they are, or how well they collaborate with patients and other colleagues.
- ❐   Above all it emphasizes only their technical accountability.

We would argue that the extent to which technical skills and scientific knowledge are considered *sufficient* analytical descriptors of all that is involved in being a surgeon, will be determined by the professional values brought up to that analysis.

A different view of all this might be that the nature of surgical practice as it is lived in reality, is complex, messy and human (what Donald Schön calls 'the swampy lowlands' of practice, as opposed to the heights of pure scientific theory). It might be seen as involving skills and scientific knowledge, but also involving activities, routines, and a wide range of other kinds of knowledge (all of which is dynamic and some of which is created in practice). Here, surgical practice is based upon human values and has complex decision-making processes and judgement at its core. Within such practice, surgeons endlessly create, negotiate and develop meanings; have to be appropriately flexible about some things and (temporarily) inflexible about others; engage all the time with multiple activities, factors and perspectives; ceaselessly formulate problems and solutions; and learn to live with the insoluble, the ephemeral, the tentative and the incomplete.

Such a practice will demand of surgeons considerable artistry, including the abilities to improvise appropriately and to draw upon insight and intuition. They will crucially be involved in adapting their knowledge and skill to individual patient care, and will bring to their practice flexibility and an open mind to continue to learn and be self-critical. They will learn from their experiences through reflection, deliberation, and investigation of their own practice. They will be prepared to confront their own attitudes, values, assumptions, beliefs and personal theories through which they see the world and within which they practice. They will engage openly with the moral and ethical dimensions of their practice. They will be meaning-makers in practice, and rounded professionals. They will expect to collaborate with patients and other colleagues, and work with, rather than on, patients. They will see themselves as professionally answerable for the whole of their conduct (not merely their skills). Only a holistic approach to teaching, learning and assessment would promote and do justice to this view, and recognize such achievements.

Clearly, it would not be possible to subscribe to both views simultaneously. They therefore provide an example of why and in what ways there can be endless contention about such matters. That is to say, what kind of a surgeon educators should seek to cultivate is a problematic matter which will need continuing review within the profession and periodic adjustment in the light of emerging developments in surgical care. And even to use the term 'cultivate' is to begin to take a particular view of what education is about. However, there has to be in a profession a broad democratic agreement on the basis of which an appropriate curriculum design can be built, which will then guide logically the teaching, learning and assessment, and to which most will subscribe for a period of time, until the need for refinement becomes clear.

It will already be clear that we subscribe to this second view, which does not deny the significance of the skills and scientific knowledge base of practice, but which sees them as necessary but by no means sufficient for cultivating a thinking surgeon, which is what we have declared from the start as our educational aim. Indeed, we are persuaded that any review of the character of professional practice needs to take account of these complexities and subtleties, these taken-for-granted elements of everyday life of professional practice as practitioners know it. We also believe that in order to plan teaching, learning and assessment for this kind of practice, practitioner-educators need to develop critical perspectives on these. We therefore summarise below what we believe about these matters. Readers are invited to use the following to clarify their own views.

We believe that professional practice:

❒   is characterized by immediate and highly informed judgements to be made, on the spot, in collaboration with fellow professionals, and made in relation to the traditional practices and values of that profession, about, and in the service of, vulnerable human beings;
❒   involves a mixture of intuition, professional on-the-spot judgement, hunch, risk-taking, and even second-guessing;

❑ is informed by esoteric and complex procedural and propositional knowledge, shaped by a recognition of the moral dimensions, controlled through the traditional professional parameters for shaping proper conduct, and influenced by the need for accountability;

❑ can be illuminated by the knowledge embedded in a piece of professional practice, but often cannot fully be expressed in words;

❑ involves creativity, and is based upon practical wisdom (which is more than mere accrued and repeated experience; it is experience reflected and deliberated upon until the deeper understanding of that practice has been achieved);

❑ cannot (except in trivial matters) be satisfactorily categorized in boxes (see for example West, (2001), and Gawande, (2001));

❑ is a lived clinical experience which is more multi-faceted than simply being about getting the patient better;

❑ is about communicating with and working with patients and colleagues, and in multi-professional teams;

❑ is about knowing and being able to assess one's own strengths and weaknesses;

❑ includes propositional (factual) medical knowledge, which is called upon in most interactions with patients, but recognizes that this kind of knowledge is often a small proportion of the whole knowledge drawn upon (see de Cossart and Fish, 2002);

❑ includes important skills of a variety of kinds.

We believe that teaching, learning and assessment should do justice to the complexities and subtleties of all this, and support learning surgeons in exploring them critically and that assessment processes should be designed to do justice to and reveal achievements in all this.

Assessment within three different models of the curriculum

Once we have begun to come to a view of the nature of the professional practice and knowledge that we wish to promote, teach and assess, we are ready to choose between the following three key models of the curriculum in order to shape the education we offer appropriately. (A curriculum contains all the details involved in a teaching programme.)

In Table 6:1, therefore, following the work of Stenhouse, we offer three ways of conceptualizing the relationship between teaching, learning and assessment (this table has been adapted from those offered in Fish, 2003; 2004; and 2005). It will be noted that the product model shows the teacher as active transmitter of knowledge, learners as passive, and assessment as often consisting only of a test at the end of the process, thus preventing it from being used as a means of teaching and learning. (This means that in a given attachment, assessment would offer a summative statement of what has been achieved, but that learners would have had only one chance to show those achievements, and no opportunity to learn from them or to show how they can develop over time). Success in such an assessment process is thought to depend on the quality of the teacher (so that the test can sometimes be considered to be a test of the teacher!). Such a model offers one way of teaching when a great deal of

Table 6:1 Three ways of seeing teaching and learning (based on the ideas of Stenhouse, 1975).

PRODUCT MODEL INTENTION	PROCESS MODEL INTENTION	RESEARCH MODEL INTENTION
teacher transmits knowledge	teacher promotes knowledge	learners explore understanding
KNOWLEDGE RESIDES IN teacher	KNOWLEDGE RESIDES IN teachers & learners	KNOWLEDGE RESIDES IN community of learners
LEARNERS ARE passive receivers of knowledge	LEARNERS ARE active seekers of knowledge	LEARNERS ARE self-aware, active learners and negotiators, who discover or reconstruct their own knowledge
(covers material fast)	(active learning takes longer)	(this takes even longer)
MOTIVATION IS VIA teacher	MOTIVATION IS VIA own active learning	MOTIVATION IS VIA group learning own active learning
SEES TEACHER AS teller/instructor who lectures and is a performer whose performance is significant in the quality of the learners' achievements	SEES TEACHER AS seeker/catalyst who facilitates learning and sets up problems to which s/he probably knows the answers but whose input does not appear to such an extent during the learning session	SEES TEACHER AS facilitator/neutral chair teacher is leader within group and learns alongside learners but only on a highly disciplined basis
SEES ASSESSMENT AS end of course tests summative teacher assessment	SEES ASSESSMENT AS part of teaching part of learning formative - and summative	SEES ASSESSMENT AS working towards self-assessment, or group assessment via formative assessment
EXAMPLES OF ASSESSMENT CRITERIA <ul><li>is accurate in replication of knowledge and skills</li><li>shows a good memory</li><li>can manipulate data as has been taught</li><li>can rehearse arguments learnt</li><li>can state issues learnt</li><li>shows required behaviour</li><li>these can be measured</li></ul>	ASSESSMENT CRITERIA <ul><li>makes personal response and shows understanding</li><li>gives evidence of thinking freshly beyond what teacher offers</li><li>can consider arguments critically</li><li>can adapt knowledge and understanding to new situations (judgement)</li><li>has sound self-knowledge</li></ul>	ASSESSMENT CRITERIA <ul><li>makes new meanings and thinks critically in new situations</li><li>can create and defend new theories rigorously</li><li>can think afresh about evidence</li><li>can select appropriately from readings and other knowledge</li><li>has sound self-knowledge</li><li>can use professional judgement</li></ul>

material has to be covered fast. The problem here, is that while it is covered by the teacher, whose presentation shows s/he knows it well, there is little opportunity either for learners to make meaning out of it for themselves, or for their teacher to know for sure whether they have received it accurately, and understood it, as opposed to merely being able to regurgitate it. A teacher who understands this can either use it only for circumstances when pure regurgitation of knowledge or learnt skills is all that is needed (as in training), or can develop approaches which to some extent can attend to these criticisms, by drawing on ideas from other models. But this will not change the fundamental mindset involved about the relationship between teaching, learning and assessment. This would be the model for a lecture programme with large numbers of learners, and/or for training people in skills which they must reproduce exactly. It would therefore suit those who wish to train surgeons as technicians.

By comparison, in the process model, the learners are more active and their knowing and understanding are facilitated by the teacher. Here, assessment is a central part of the teaching and learning, feeding into an on-going understanding of the learner's achievements, which is instrumental in shaping the next activities of both teacher and learner (is formative). These on-going assessments ultimately offer a pattern of evidence *across* the period of learning, which will provide a robust and fair summative statement about what learners have achieved and how they have developed. This model can be caricatured as 'discovery learning' which implies that teachers often set simulated problems as a means to an end which they do not fully declare. It does not, of course, have to be used in that way, and it would seem to lend itself to the active learning needed by professionals as pro-active learners in clinical settings. However, it does not free them from their teachers' views and values, may not emancipate them from their own earlier mindset, and may not enable them to see the world in new ways.

A third view of the relationship between teaching and learning places the onus on the learners as understanding and achieving within their own negotiated agenda. This makes the teachers' role that of one learning resource among many, and sees assessment as developing self-knowledge and success in investigative approaches to learning. However, it can be caricatured as directionless activity which is offered by teachers who do not know what they are doing and who let learners engage in a free-for-all. In fact, this model could provide learners in clinical settings with the real richness of challenge and opportunity that education should provide.

Of course, it should be remembered that models are simplistic and reductionist, and that each merely offers a way of thinking which will be useful for different educational intentions. These models are only a guide and the educator must choose appropriately. Such a decision cannot be shaped by idealistic views but by the current context and state of educational development. In reality at the moment, we believe that the research model is probably too far removed from where education for the profession of surgery currently stands to make it a viable basis for planning teaching and learning in surgery (though its educational approach might prove useful as a longer-term ambition). We also see the product model as one way of thinking about 'covering content', but as leading to a narrow, skills-based approach in practical teaching and learning in clinical settings. So, we conclude that the process model currently provides the best basis for cultivating a thinking surgeon.

Given the popularity of competency-based approaches to assessment and the almost ubiquitous muddling of competence and competencies, which are in fact two very different concepts, we now offer the vital distinctions between them, as a further set of arguments for eschewing the skills-based, technician view of surgical education.

The vital distinction between competence and competencies

The *competency-based approach* to training believes that all that is needed in preparing for practice as a professional is a collection of all the skills (*competencies*) that can be listed as used in that job. We believe (in common with other educational thinkers like Broadfoot, 1993 and 2000; David Carr, 1993; Wilf Carr, 1995; Eraut, 1994; Golby and Parrott, 1999; Talbot, 2004; White and Stancombe, 2003; and Wragg, 1994), that this is a naïve and rather tired and inappropriate approach to preparing professionals for practice. We see it as rooted in a generally impoverished, worryingly values free, and morally bankrupt view of teaching, learning and assessment, which is concerned only with training people in skills that cash out into visible behaviour whose measurement is deemed to provide satisfactory evidence of capability to work as a professional.

The current obsession with measurement rejects the importance of anything to which numbers cannot easily be accorded, and therefore ignores all the crucial elements that drive visible behaviour in the professional (like moral awareness and professional judgement). In a competency-based course, teaching and learning is seen in terms of an industrial transaction where what is important is what will conduce to the efficient and cheap delivery of a product. In this view, assessment becomes a simplistic and narrow activity. It places emphasis on visible skills (that may hide quite other views); overlooks, and thus leads to an erosion of, professional values like sensitivity and imagination; ignores the moral issues of how, when and where such skills should and should not be used; and inculcates an inflexibility which mitigates against future development (particularly professional self-development).

In the competency-based approach, the occupational skills needed within a job are listed and categorized, as a means of Quality Assurance. As Fish, 1991 pointed out, this was about quality in manufacturing industries, who in Britain had to conform to British Standard 5750, which gave 19 criteria a company should use in deciding how to operate quality assurance. The skills are thus turned into competencies and used as the means of assessing performance in the workplace. This has been of particular use in Further Education and associated with vocational training leading to National Vocational Qualifications (NVQs), which were set up by the Government Training Agency (see, for example, Burke, 1989; and Wolf, 1995). It is arguable, however, that clinical practice for postgraduate doctors is rather different from the workplace inhabited by school leavers with NVQs. The implication here is that everyone in the workplace can be 'standardized' against this perfected list. There will never be universal agreement about exactly how many skills are necessary, even for the simplest of jobs, let alone in surgery. For example a key problem is that such a list can ramify endlessly. Other problems include the following.

- ❐ How and from where can such skills be derived? (On what basis will they be chosen?).
- ❐ How explicitly and in what detail should they be defined? (Ever greater detail is always a temptation).
- ❐ How many should there be? (There will always be an impetus to list yet more).
- ❐ What will count as evidence for their acquisition? (How many times must they be demonstrated before they are deemed to be acquired?).
- ❐ Will learners need to pass them all, and should they pass each at the same level?
- ❐ What order of priority (weighting) will they be given, and how?
- ❐ How will length of experience affect the level expected?

We do not wish to undervalue skills. Competencies may be necessary, but for us they will never be a sufficient base for the education of members of a profession. Indeed, we suspect that those who - mostly unthinkingly - embrace the competency-based approach to professional education (or worse, who use the terms 'competency' or 'competencies' as if they mean the same as 'competence'), are not aware of the underlying values of, and crucial issues which arise within, this view of professional practice. Sadly, we are aware of a number of Department of Health documents which use these terms interchangeably. Further, we suspect that there will be no richness of educational development in health care until these matters are properly and openly debated and the real 'lived' values of professions are genuinely expressed in appropriate educational aims and processes.

By contrast, a professional's *competence* is concerned with an holistic notion of professional practice, and the assessment of this is based upon judgements of quality (Eraut, 1998, p. 128), where what is important is the 'ability to perform the tasks and roles required to the expected standard' (Eraut, 1998, p.129). He also makes the point that: 'what is to count as competence results from negotiations, explicit or implicit, between employers, professionals and clients' (to which he also adds, professional bodies, educational providers and the government). This means that it is incumbent upon professionals to be articulate about the distinction between competence and competencies, and be clear about what they see as appropriate for their profession.

The idea of competence (which being holistic, *does not have a plural version*) is concerned with placing the necessary skills of professional practice into a wider context which takes account of the essence and core of what is really involved in being a professional. It recognizes that professionals engage in intelligent and wise conduct, rather than trained behaviour, use professional judgement rather than following protocols, and draw on knowledge in creative ways rather than simply applying it unthinkingly to practice. Within this, it recognizes the significance of skills, but sees that they alone are not sufficient as the content for teaching and assessing professionals, and that knowing where, how and why to use (or not use) these skills creatively in new circumstances is the central issue for those who work on a daily basis with individual patients and clients whose needs are all different.

We believe, (with Eraut, 1998), that competency-based training may be useful for preparing people to enter an occupation where routine performance is all that matters, but is inappropriate as the basis for preparing people for a profession where complex clinical thinking, knowing and doing all have to be shaped to the particular issues raised by each individual case. This means that professionals need to learn how to practise by drawing upon all these matters, need to understand the complex relationships between them, and need to explore how to bring theory into relationship with practice. By contrast, in an occupation, practice is not simply of prime importance, it is the *only* important focus. There, theory (of any kind) is not regarded as of any significance. Rather what matters most in training for the job, is mastering specific and standardized skills and demonstrating that mastery to the same level in every situation.

Given the above, the reader may be left wondering how competency-based assessment has been permitted to be imposed on professional education. We believe that this is probably because of failure to distinguish between competence and competencies, and the lack of clarity about the vital distinctions between these similar looking and sounding words. The difference between words is not mere semantics, it reflects crucially different views of the world.

The work of David Carr illustrates how the confusion may have occurred, and then demonstrates how the resulting confusion can be unravelled. He shows that 'competence', the wider and more holistic term, is understood to refer to wide capacities which we use thoughtfully and which 'entail the voluntary and deliberate exercise of principled judgement in the light of rational knowledge and understanding' (see D. Carr, 1993, p. 257). He makes the point that competence is the result of education. By contrast, competencies refers only to a narrower, more atomistic view of practice and these could be understood in the dispositional sense. Dispositions include skills, faculties, habits and are caused by innate ability or training, which 'leans us' in the direction of using them without ever thinking about them. He indicates that it is easy to relate and confuse the two (particularly when the term 'competent' is used in both categories), but that for the preparation of professionals it is vital to hold them apart. Clearly, there is a world of difference between, on the one hand, work as characterizable in terms of pre-specifiable discrete itemised skills (competencies) and which is all about visible behaviour, and on the other hand that which is described as conduct resulting from an educated understanding (competence).

The two aspects of competence, as David Carr goes on to show, clearly ought to go together, and we would wish to see competencies as a part of this whole which is referred to as competence. We have to be careful in assessing them. Achievement in competencies alone, which looks like sound practice, does not in fact guarantee either a sound underpinning understanding or an ability to develop in the longer term. For example, a trained practitioner who is under observation (assessment), may perform on the surface routinely well at a given level. But this does not guarantee real commitment to that behaviour or a principled understanding of it, and does not ensure any basis for further development. On the other hand, an educated practitioner, who might perform badly on an (assessment) occasion in terms of dispositional effectiveness but who is able to reflect upon practice, will be able to improve and develop that practice continuously (see also Fish, 1995; and Fish and Twinn, 1997).

Table 6.2 offers a representation of how to tease these two concepts apart.

Table 6:2 The vital distinction between competence and competencies (based on the ideas of Carr, 1993).

Competence as a holistic notion	Competencies as skills
The term 'competent' can be used in both categories, but means something very different in each:	
competent meaning showing overall competence	competent meaning shows a competency and/or competencies
An example would be:	An example would be:
X is the more competent of these two doctors	Y is a competent shot
(meaning: X's overall competence shows as the ability to conduct him/herself and his/her work in different ways on different occasions according to what the situation demands)	(meaning: Y always operates using the same skills efficiently, and in the same way wherever s/he is, and is never tempted to alter his/her approach whatever happens)
This is about overall competence - seen as holistic	This is about narrow atomistic skills, habits, mechanical efficiency
- a label for the capacity to operate skills in a thoughtful manner	- a label for a particular ability which is reliable and unchanging under all circumstances
Here, competent means someone has a capacity to operate successfully as a result of using their knowledge and skills flexibly (shaped by education)	Here, competent means someone has a disposition (has been shaped) to respond reliably and always in the same way (shaped by training or by being born thus)
Exercising a capacity means a voluntary and deliberate exercise of principled judgement in the light of rational knowledge and understanding	Exercising a disposition means using inherent tendencies which enable agents to perform certain specifiable functions either by training or natural endowment
Here, the competent person is autonomous - a free agent whose aspiration/deliberate achievement is gained in the light of knowledge and standards	Here, the competent person has ability, power, effectiveness formed in him/her (by nature or training). Here, competency has been caused!
Here, conduct is rationally ordered according to reason and principle	Here, behaviour is controlled by routine and reliability in that skill
We choose to exercise our capacity	Our dispositions exercise us
Here, the competent person is acting in a broadly principled or reflective and informed way - and has to be judged on the basis of whether the principles were sound and the actions were moral and achieved their intentions	Here, the competent person is acting well, efficiently and effectively according to some verifiable canon or acceptable standard of performance (the same for all circumstances)

The competency-based approach may be summarised as follows. It:

- ❏ may improve some basic skills in the short term (though possibly at the expense of rigidity in the longer term);
- ❏ is readily organised into a bureaucratic model for administrative purposes, thus apparently increasing efficiency (and actually increasing bureaucratic control!);
- ❏ appears to lead to objective assessment of practice (though such apparent objectivity only hides further value judgements!);
- ❏ is about improving performance (perhaps at the expense of understanding);
- ❏ undervalues theory and research;
- ❏ has no interest in theorizing about practice;
- ❏ has no interest in the moral and ethical dimensions of professional practice;
- ❏ offers professionals no inbuilt means of developing and refining practice;
- ❏ embraces the idea that professionalism can be judged only against the notion of fitness for purpose (ensures that the ends are never challenged);
- ❏ emphasizes the acquisition of basic skills at the expense of developing understanding, refining practical theoretical knowledge and engaging in scholarly activity;
- ❏ is interested in behaviour which is visible but not conduct which acknowledges the moral and ethical values, beliefs and theories which drive action;
- ❏ recognizes the need for professionals to be technically accountable (but not more than this);
- ❏ arises from a deficit model of professionalism;
- ❏ values:
  - certainties about the knowledge, skills and strategies to be a successful professional;
  - being able to analyse skills and the main characteristics of a professional down to the finest detail and being able to observe these as visible behaviour;
  - setting basic standards against which everything can be judged;
  - training;
  - measuring observable behaviour as a simple route to increasing efficiency;
  - the language and ideas of managerialism and of industrial output as equally appropriate to discussing professionalism.

By contrast, the competence approach values:

- ❏ professional practice as involving open capacities which cannot be mastered;
- ❏ professional judgement and its complexity (the ability to choose between competing priorities, values, actions, interpretations);
- ❏ the complex and uncertain nature of day-to-day practice;
- ❏ professionals' moral responsibility to vulnerable patients/clients, and colleagues, and in addition, professional answerability in respect of their technical proficiency;
- ❏ the ability to utilize general knowledge, thinking and doing (which includes skills but far more) so that it is shaped to the specific and particular individual needs of patients;

❑ the development of a (personal) principled base from which to practise as a professional;

❑ an understanding of the importance of values and self-knowledge in respect of the individual's professional values;

❑ the need to attend to the moral and ethical dimensions of practice;

❑ an understanding of the wider issues of professionalism and the responsibilities of being a member of a profession;

❑ the use of a range of skills and of the importance of choosing rationally between them;

❑ self-knowledge and the ability of a professional to attend to their own professional development;

❑ the ability to influence key decisions at the level of policy and the capacity to take an active role in the development of the profession itself.

Equipped with an educational philosophy (an understanding of the choices available and the reasons for choosing the broader rather than the narrower approaches to education in general and assessment in particular), the surgical teacher and learner can now turn to the practical aspects of assessment of the learning surgeon in clinical settings.

What should be assessed in surgical practice and by what means?

What should be assessed in the clinical setting to educate thinking surgeons?

We see the following as needing to be attended to by learning surgeons through teaching and assessment in the clinical setting (the fine detail of how they can be taught and assessed within surgical practice is the substance of Part two of this book):

❑ medical and surgical theory (all theoretical factual knowledge relevant to practice);

❑ educational processes (how to learn in clinical settings, how to reflect on practice);

❑ the principles of clinical practice;

❑ the principles of technical and operative procedures and how to learn them;

❑ the principles of clinical processes and how to learn them;

❑ the skills of clinical and surgical practices, as specific to the specialty;

❑ the specialty-specific knowledge that lies beneath and drives clinical/surgical practice;

❑ the clinical thinking that lies beneath surgical and clinical practice;

❑ professionalism and ability to communicate and work within a multi-professional team.

❑ self-knowledge and an understanding of personal limitations as well as abilities;

❑ a knowledge of appropriate and relevant research, how to critique it, and under what circumstances it will be relevant to given cases;

❑ the use made of all learning opportunities.

It is interesting to reflect that very little of this would be appropriately evidenced and documented via ticked boxes.

Special note

It should be noted that we do not use the terms 'generic skills' and 'generic clinical processes', that are common to many current curriculum documents. This is deliberate. We recognize that it flies in the face of current practice for medicine and surgery but we do not subscribe either to the idea that skills are all that is involved in any doctor/patient interaction or to the notion that skills that can be learnt in one context will directly transfer to another. Indeed, we roundly refute such assumptions. Even activities and interactions which seem to crop up in every medical context (like doctors simply introducing themselves to patients or breaking bad news) have to be extensively adapted, re-adjusted and actually replaced by other skills in different contexts. How a doctor introduces him/herself in a psychiatric ward would be different in kind as well as in process and skills from the self-introduction made in an orthopaedic practice. Learning to break bad news and gain consent for treatment in an HIV clinic is fundamentally different from gaining consent for an HIV test as a routine matter of differential diagnosis for a patient within a medical ward. Crucially it is and should be a different experience for each patient. We conclude, therefore, that it is not the detail of skills, processes and procedures that are generic and thus travel. Rather, it is *principles* that can be transferred and used in all contexts. This is why we have, throughout this book, so stressed the importance of principles and of having a principled approach to practice.

We therefore turn now to establishing a principled approach to assessment.

The principles that should guide that assessment

The detail of using assessment in the clinical setting must be left to the surgeon educator and the learning surgeon. But this educational transaction needs to be guided by and grounded in sound principles. Indeed, any system of assessment must be coherent and principled. The following are offered, for critique, as examples of the most useful key principles for enacting assessment in clinical settings in all professions.

- ❐ Assessment should always be a learning experience and centred first on facilitating learning.
- ❐ Its purpose(s) should be clear and educational and understood by all involved.
- ❐ It should be carried out in practice by those who teach the learner in the practice setting (though they can also include an external assessor as well).
- ❐ Criteria should be clear and understood by all involved.
- ❐ Assessment should assess that which it says it does.
- ❐ The elements to be assessed must be derived from the aims of the overall educational programme and the intentions of the individual learner and teacher.
- ❐ Observation should be systematic, rigorous and take account of the complexities of practice.
- ❐ Approaches to assessment that go beyond mere observation should be developed.

- ❒ Evidence - of a variety of kinds - should be carefully recorded and utilized.
- ❒ Multiple perspectives should be taken (assessment should be of a variety of elements of practice, and should call upon at least three assessors to do justice to the three-dimensional nature of clinical practice).
- ❒ The role of professional judgement should not be under-valued.
- ❒ Simple negative inferences should never be drawn from negative situations, without first checking on how the learner construed the situation (and even the purpose of assessment) in the first place.
- ❒ What counts as evidence needs to be carefully thought through and agreed by assessor and assessee.
- ❒ Learners' achievements should be seen and reported as outcomes of the interaction between the context and the learner. (The learner can only show surgical capabilities within what the attachment provides.)
- ❒ In all assessments (formative and summative; formal and informal) the following information should be taken account of, through multiple perspectives on the learner's progress:
  - the visible elements of the learner's performance;
  - the impact of that performance on all others involved;
  - the learner's ideas, beliefs, values, assumptions, beneath the surface of performance;
  - the formal theoretical dimensions drawn upon by the learner during practice;
  - how the learner has related theory and practice;
  - the learner's ability to theorize their own practice;
  - how the learner has capitalized on the learning opportunities provided;
  - the learner's self-knowledge;
  - how much input there has been from the teacher;
  - how the resulting assessment judgements cross check with those made of the learner by others.

The presence of multiple perspectives on the learner's achievements in complex practice settings means that *interpretation* of the assessment evidence is necessary. The soundness of the assessment is therefore related to the rigour with which those multiple perspectives are collected, recorded and utilized. Thus, in all these issues, in the end, the teacher/assessor's professional judgement has to be employed alongside the range of evidence available.

What are the key elements of assessment for surgeons?

The bases on which assessment should be designed

Defining and agreeing the purpose of assessment is therefore a vital starting point for surgical educators. The answers to the following questions should be driven by a clear educational philosophy in which facilitating the progress of the learning surgeon is the central concern, where a partnership in learning between teacher and learner is valued, and where the learning environment nurtures the learner. The latter will be the result of a balance between challenge and comfort that is appropriate for that learner.

- ❑ What is assessment for? (What do you value assessment for?).
- ❑ Who is it for?
- ❑ How does it relate to learning?
- ❑ When, in time, in relation to learning, should it happen, and why?

The choices available to someone designing assessment include:

- ❑ formal/informal; final/continuous; external/internal; convergent/divergent;
- ❑ summative (at the end of the learning)/formative (integral to it);
- ❑ quantitative (producing numbers for items)/qualitative (about understanding the learner);
- ❑ objectivity/subjectivity (some argue there is no such thing as objectivity);
- ❑ criterion referenced (criteria or competencies as standard)/ norm referenced (average as standard or curve of distribution as standard);
- ❑ format for assessment: written/performance/oral/video/profile/portfolio/diary.

Each choice made about the above expresses a particular sense of educational purpose, and will exclude some other possibilities. Formal assessment should never rest on a one-off process. It is about looking at the learner's achievements and progress and should be designed to help shape further teaching and learning. The learner's ability to learn should be considered during the assessment. All assessment should seek to develop the learner's ability to self-assess.

The gate-keeping process

Progression from being a learning surgeon to entering a career post is the aim of programmes of training in surgery. Evidence that the individual has achieved the standards set at key points along the programme is mandatory. At the end of the programme there must be a summative process that brings together all the evidence and recognizes the learner's success (or otherwise) in the whole programme.

Once the assessments within an individual attachment have been rigorously carried out, and have fed into a summative process for that attachment, they can also be used summatively for gate-keeping purposes to provide evidence that the learner is ready to progress beyond the programme. Key means of establishing rigour involve cross-checking the evidence and judgements made. As each assessment of the learner is compared against the next, evidence of progress is what should be sought. At summative assessment, larger patterns of development should be sought, but this too is a complex matter, requiring a recognition of the balance of different purposes of assessment and different ways of looking at criteria. Further, assessors need to remember that virtually all research into learning has taught us that it happens in fits and starts, involves plateaux of various kinds (which are actually important in the learning process), and that it does not proceed incrementally, in a simplistic way.

The gate-keeping process also needs to take account of both the learner's overt achievements, and the use made of the learning opportunities. This will enable important distinctions to be made between someone who is a quite good performer naturally, but who hasn't bothered to use the new opportunities to learn (and who may not be a learner), and someone who has struggled a little more, but who is actually a better bet as a professional practitioner in the longer term. Thus, assessment is both about achievements in surgery and in the process of learning itself. Once surgeon educators understand these educational matters they will not need to be taught anything further about the gate-keeping aspects of assessment, and they will certainly not need to have public money poured into assessment training.

Ensuring the standards of good surgical practice

Good assessment will develop the understanding of surgeons about what is necessary to meet the standards set by the regulatory body, the GMC. Standards set in isolation from such understanding will lack depth and true purpose.

The GMC first produced *Good Medical Practice* in 1992. Its seven key points not only serve as a framework for Trust appraisal of all members of the profession of medicine, but are also being used to develop curricula for the education and training of new doctors. The RCS Eng responded to this with *Good Surgical Practice*, recently revised in 2002. This sets standards more specifically for surgical as distinct from medical practice.

The RCS Eng's curriculum framework for the first three years of surgical training (currently SHOs) sets out surgical values which have been developed by practising surgeons. These values are to be part of the educational development of new surgeons. A mapping exercise has demonstrated that these values underpin the seven elements of *Good Medical Practice* and *Good Surgical Practice*.

Two key problems for the assessment of surgeons in the clinical setting

If good education in clinical settings needs to reflect the true complexity of both the nature of clinical practice and the nature of clinical knowledge, then the assessments we carry out must do justice to this. We have recognized that many important elements that drive our professional practice lie beneath its surface. But two key questions emerge:

☐   How shall we reveal them?
☐   How shall we assess them?

We believe that there are three important aspects of our practice that drive our surface actions and conduct, and that this is so whether or not they lie tacit within our practice or are explicitly recognized. These are:

1.   that which lurks beneath the iceberg of professional practice (our theories, beliefs, assumptions, and values);

2.   the knowledge we draw on while we are 'doing'; and
3.   the thinking we are engaging in while we are 'doing'.

These three 'drivers' of professional practice powerfully affect conduct in clinical settings. Awareness and refinement of them will shape the practitioner's success with patients in ways far beyond what can be achieved by learning and deploying skills alone. Patients themselves are often very aware and quick to recognize this. They read the values, beliefs and assumptions of their doctors in the way those doctors conduct themselves in their interaction with them. This radically affects how far they trust the knowledge, thinking and doing of those doctors.

The refinement of these three highly significant drivers depends upon the ability to surface them, and examine them. Their significance for overall success as a doctor or surgeon also means that it is important to assess them. Clearly, ticked boxes will not be sufficient. We believe that the key means to this is reflective practice that is shaped to focus sharply and educationally on these drivers of practice. The detail of this is explored both in the next chapter and throughout Part two of this book.

Documenting assessment

It is for the above reasons that we regard the tick-box approach to assessment of doctors generally and surgeons specifically as insufficient. We accept, as does Eraut, that the public would be 'distinctly uneasy if evidence of authentic performance did not play a major part in the assessment of professional competence' (Eraut, 1998, p. 135). But the development and refinement of conduct depends upon drivers like those we have listed above. Their development is what affects the development of clinical practice. The documentation of evidence of achievement in the clinical setting needs to attend to this, and the development of practitioners as researchers of their own practice also depends upon such documentation. We therefore believe that beyond the tick boxes (which convey small and ambiguous details) we need to develop the use of: reflective accounts of practice; narratives of practitioner development; and even recordings of practice, together with proper critiques of these. For the detail of this, see the final chapter of this book.

It is customary for those who wish to deflect these ideas or avoid engaging in these complex practices, to argue that there is a danger of breaching confidentiality and of fuelling litigation in all this. Naturally, proper research ethics need to be adopted in relation to narratives and other accounts, and they need to be kept confidentially and only the insights shared (see Chapter 11, which provides details of how to access the full ethics associated with educational research). Without this possibility there will be no development. We therefore do not find these arguments persuasive.

The educational portfolio described in the GPPS curriculum framework is an example of how the overall evidence of achievement within an attachment can be documented. In various sections of the portfolio the elements that make up a learning surgeon's achievements in clinical practice can be documented. If the principles of assessment listed above are applied to this

Table 6:3 The key sections of the GPPS portfolio.

Section of portfolio	Contents	Elements assessed
Introduction	Personal details	Professional values
Section 1	Agreed aims for attachment	Overview of learning intentions for attachment
Section 2	Specialty monitoring technical/operative record sheets	Overview of operative opportunities
Section 3	Triggered assessment forms and generic technical operative skills record sheets	Specialty-specific operative skills; generic theoretical knowledge; generic educational processes; generic technical/operative skills; specialty-specific theoretical knowledge
Section 4	Generic clinical processes forms	Generic clinical processes
Section 5	Reflective journal statement	Development of generic theoretical knowledge; development of generic educational processes; development of professional values
Section 6	Research experience statement	Development of knowledge and experience of a range of enquiry processes, and evaluation of research evidence
Section 7	Summative assessment and MRCS achievements	Overall progress in practical and theoretical elements - both at the end of each attachment and at the end of the SHO experience. (Generic theoretical and clinical knowledge, and communication skills assessed in MRCS)
Appendix	Log of operations	(Provides overview of operative experience)

kind of repository of evidence, then it will be a principled and valuable document capable of shaping future learning as well as recording past successes. It will only be so, however, if the teacher and the learner value it as such a resource and keep it up-to-date.

Professional judgement, assessment and level of supervision

We have already alluded to the fact that consultants have been engaged in the assessment of surgeons for many decades, and that in all cases their professional judgement is an inevitable part of that process, determining for example, the interpretations of conduct, the choices made about the level of performance, and decisions made about the level of future supervision needed as a learner progresses through the system.

We do not argue for this use of professional judgement to change, but for it to be better recognized as a proper part of this process. While such judgements must be principled, and backed up by evidence, no additional training is required for surgeons to be able to do this. Rather, they need to understand the matters we have offered in this chapter. As with their clinical professional judgement, of course, their educational professional judgement will develop and be refined *in practice*. This will happen in the community of assessment practice in which surgeon educators engage. (We have already argued for the principles of multiple perspectives in assessment, which themselves will contribute to the refinement of the assessment process.)

Validity and reliability

Whenever there is discussion of the assessment of surgeons in the clinical setting, there are calls to prevent this from happening until the process recommended can be 'proved' to be valid and reliable. There are several deeply serious misunderstandings beneath this reaction. One is the mistaken belief that any system of assessment is able to be perfected. The second is that education is a science and must be treated like one, and that science has the only means of proof and of ensuring validity and reliability.

Of course, educational activities like assessment and research can be made reliable and valid, but anyone seeking to do so in scientific terms, or who thinks that only science has the processes for this, will inevitably fail. This is because assessment is a form of educational inquiry, and education as a discipline has its own means of attending to these matters. It uses qualitative research procedures to investigate the complexity of lived experience, within which there are processes for ensuring the reliability and validity of both the process and the product. These processes take proper and rigorous account of the nature of educational practice and have been developed and refined within the research community of educational practitioners, of which the British Educational Research Association (BERA) is the leading body.

Reliability here means the assessment process will assess that which it sets out to do, and not, (by accident), some other element. This involves teacher and learner being clear about and agreeing what is being assessed and how, and how these are appropriate to the context chosen for the assessment. The reliability of the product of assessment depends on showing that the same process can (at the level of principle) produce the same result across multiple instances. Several formative assessment results thus need to feed into the summative and final assessment.

Validity here means checking that a variety of assessment processes are used both within the assessment of a practical process and across the practice as a whole and that these do justice to its complexity and are represented in the final assessment. This involves the use of multiple perspectives (sometimes also called triangulation).

Before turning to the second part of this book, we provide a résumé of our argument so far, and look at its implications for working in the current context of surgical practice.

From apprentice to professional: turning training into medical education

Introduction

Key issues emerging from Part one

The problems that this leaves us with

How to turn competency-based requirements for training into education

A concrete example

Introduction

In this résumé we highlight and bring together an overview of the key educational arguments of Part one and consider their implications for current practice in Post Graduate Medical and Dental Education (PGMDE) generally and surgery in particular. We conclude from our arguments that the education of doctors and surgeons is preferable to training them in skills. However, current government requirements, (as for example in F2), being based upon competencies and on the notion of simple forms of training and assessment, do not provide a congenial foundation for the education of a thinking surgeon. Further, we fear other curricula as they emerge will be seduced away from broader educational goals to follow an easy but ultimately fruitless approach to curriculum development, based only upon competencies. Accordingly, we provide some principles to work on in order to engage in educational practice of the kind we discuss in Part one, whilst conforming as required to these narrower intentions. We end this résumé with a concrete example.

Key issues emerging from Part one

Our early arguments in Part one claimed the need for PGMDE to cultivate a mindful professional rather than produce an efficient apprentice. We argued for the cultivation of thinking surgeons (who have all the craft skills but seat them in a broader understanding of surgical and professional practice), rather than technical craftspersons, whose skills are their only asset. We showed that (particularly in the 21st Century with all its constraints on practising in the clinical setting), it is now crucial to go beyond apprenticeship (with its overtones of simple training) and to develop a richer approach to the professional education of surgeons.

We pointed out that training (which is concerned to bring about a change in visible behaviour) takes an essentially technical rational and unproblematic view of the learner and of learning. It is suitable for changing behaviour only where no deep thought needs to be associated with actions (as in a factory worker). By contrast, the practice of education recognizes that everything about education, being values based, is complex, contestable, and problematic, but that this is a more suitable approach to developing the work of practising professionals who are already postgraduates and whose employment in the clinical setting involves coping with complex clinical cases. We concluded that complex as educational practice is, it is the only approach that is seriously suitable for this purpose.

We said that this is about the need to educate the whole professional who accordingly treats the patient holistically, rather than training a technician who will be more inclined to deal with the immediately relevant component parts of a body. The crucial distinction here is between a professional who has overall competence (at his/her level of practice), and one who has only been trained in competencies (a series of discrete skills). We pointed out that beneath the surface and visible behaviour of a professional, lies a number of important elements which need to be recognized as seriously affecting that practice. These are elements associated with the expected conduct of members of a profession and the more personal assumptions, beliefs, theories and values that shape a professional's actions. Such actions are also underpinned by his/her thinking and knowing, and by a recognition of the complex ethical and moral issues associated with working with patients who by definition are vulnerable.

These are all powerful drivers of a professional's practice, but training does not attend to them. It gives no guarantee that the changes it produces in behaviour will be more than cosmetic. It alters the surface but produces mere conformation to requirements, which may only be engaged in to please the assessor during the observation, and may afterwards be abandoned. It attends only to the changes needed immediately, provides no means for on-going self-development, and provokes the need for retraining whenever further changes are needed, together with endless inspection to ensure conformity. By contrast, to educate professionals by helping them to recognize, understand and develop all the elements that come together in their practice, is to produce a thinking practitioner who will develop or change their behaviour in the light of their new understanding. Such understanding develops commitment to refine, develop or change action. This means that a professional can be self-directing, use discretion and be self-supervising. Training provides short-term fixes but at a high ultimate cost. We have argued that Britain currently cannot afford to spend its resources on training rather than educating surgeons.

Given that much of what an educator attends to (or rather enables the learner to attend to), is invisible and therefore difficult to capture and also to assess, we argued for the recognition of the central role in education of rigorous investigative reflection on practice. Reflection, we argued, needs to be shared in both spoken and written form, will allow learners to make their own sense of their own practice, and enable teachers to begin to understand where learners are in this process. The evidence from this formative assessment can be used at summative points, so that the role of reflection in assessment is also crucial.

The problems that this leaves us with

The practice of education, then, is arguably more suitable to the cultivation of a thinking surgeon than training in competencies. There are two problems associated with this. The first is that, so far as we can ascertain, the voice of education has not yet contributed to the decision-making about curricula for PGMDE, (and so this book is an attempt to set out the arguments for education rather than training). The second is that training is now the required process for postgraduate doctors, and, as a consequence much activity within PGMDE is focused upon developing the assessment of competencies. This is given further thrust by the ubiquity of competency-based curricula throughout health care. (It should be noted though, that professionals who have grown up through this process are mainly wedded to protocols and do not take the final responsibility for vital medical decisions in cases of complex care.) It also seems to be the case that the climate in which doctors are developed in the clinical setting seems more conducive to the short-term approach that training provides, though it is only a quick fix response to a deeper problem.

How to turn competency-based requirements for training into education

Since we are suggesting that training, whilst necessary, is not sufficient, and that, in principle, all education must start where the learner is (which in a training mode is preset by current requirements), it seems to us that the way forward is to clarify what training can achieve, and then supplement it with ideas and processes that will provide what is sufficient to enable it to be counted as the practice of education.

Training, then, attends to teaching and assessing skills. Training is concerned with 'generic skills', and with maintaining as simple as possible an approach to what needs to be learnt.

What training does not do is as follows.

- ❏ It does not raise issues about the ends to which these skills need to be employed, nor is it overly concerned with the overall goal for PGMDE, assuming the enterprise to be simple, and the end product of technical expertise (and the means to achieving this) to be unproblematic.
- ❏ It does not hold as significant the specific context in which the skills are learnt and assessed, skills being seen as simply transferable. (This is a notion we reject because skills cannot be learnt and applied directly in all practice irrespective of the context. We believe that only principles are generic.)
- ❏ It does not take a holisitic approach to the development of the practitioner, or medicine, or the patient.
- ❏ It does not attend to the importance of conduct by a member of a profession.
- ❏ It does not attend to what drives professional actions as illustrated in the iceberg of professional practice.
- ❏ It does not attend to the thinking that drives a professional's actions, decisions and professional judgements.
- ❏ It therefore lacks an ethical and moral dimension.
- ❏ It does not attend to the knowledge that underlies the skills a professional uses.

❐　It does not help learners to make their own sense of their experiences.

❐　It does not attend to assessment other than by tick-boxes.

The practice of education can embed all these missing matters into and around the training process and its associated assessment procedures. It can thus ensure that the skills being learnt are properly related to real practice. The practice of education can:

❐　set skills training inside carefully articulated goals of education which relate to understanding and to the holisitic work of the practitioner;

❐　teach and assess the individual skills within a properly contextualized individual situation;

❐　teach and assess the skills in such a way that they are seen as part of the holistic resources of the practitioner;

❐　relate the skills to the wider requirements made on practitioners resulting from their membership of a profession;

❐　make visible the underlying values, beliefs, assumptions and theories of the individual professional so that they are aware of them and can develop them;

❐　make explicit the knowledge that underpins the practitioner's doing;

❐　make explicit the thinking that underpins the skills (including the practitioner's decision-making and professional judgement);

❐　consider explicitly the moral and ethical dimensions arising from the specific context in which the skills are taught and assessed;

❐　use rigorous reflection on practice to enable the learner to make greater meaning out of the experience and to demonstrate the evidence of these achievements.

A concrete example

We have recently been involved in the development for surgical SHOs of a programme for preparing First Assistants in theatre. This has evolved from an in-house training initiative for senior nurses and other suitable professionals. The training consisted mainly of a list of eleven skills, which learners had to get signed off by consultant surgeons or other senior staff, as they demonstrated they could carry them out in real practice. The senior nurse responsible for the programme had already surrounded these bald skills with: a list of knowledge which should accompany the use of the skill; a demand for some reflection on those skills; and a requirement for learners to comment in writing on how confident they felt about using them in similar settings.

The list of skills is as follows: pre-operative assessment; positioning of patient; skin preparation; draping the patient prior to surgery; assisting with haemostasis; handling of instruments including camera holding for minimal invasive surgery; handling and retracting tissue and organs; assisting with cutting sutures; performing skin closure by suture and clips; application of dressing to the wound; transfer of patient to anaesthetic care unit/recovery.

The original paperwork for the assessment of these skills was similar for each skill and Table R:1 outlines that which guided the assessment of the first of these skills.

Table R:1 The original competency-based form for the assessment of First Assistants as related to the first skill.

Number 1 assessment	Component elements of the skill Pre-operative	N	A	C B	P	E	Self-assessment date and signature	Assessor date and signature
Skills	Identification of patient history in relationship to pending operative procedure							
	Manner and ability of questioning and listening							
	Interpretation of these for managing possible care intra-operatively							
	Setting up suitable objectives for post-operative care							
	Communication with other members of multidisciplinary team							
	Awareness of necessary record keeping							
Knowledge	**Key points within the elements**							
	Demonstrate communication techniques							
	Show an awareness of tools for adequate communication							
	Demonstrate knowledge of operative procedures							
	Demonstrate the Nursing Code for record keeping (2002)							

Standard Required

The objectives are: to undertake this task competently, knowing who should undergo pre-operative assessment and when and where it should take place; to incorporate knowledge based on possible facts supporting this, identifying risks, benefits and informed consent; to demonstrate a suitable level of communication skills; and to recognise the need for accurate record keeping.

Student self-assessment of this skill

Do you have complete understanding of how you are meant to incorporate this skill into everyday practice?	YES / NO
Are there any aspects of this skill in which you feel you need further practice or assistance?	YES / NO
Do you feel competent in this skill to:	
1. perform the skill unassisted	YES / NO
2. perform the skill unsupervised	YES / NO
3. teach the skill to another student	YES / NO
What extra help would assist you in improving your competence in this skill?	

We took this and adapted it for doctors, where the competencies were not a major requirement. This led to the production of the following form.

Table R:2 The SHOs record of learning for the First Assistant Programme as related to the first skill.

1. Pre-operative/diagnostic assessment		Date: …………………………………		
Context for assessment:		Specific case:		
1. Knowledge	I verify that I know: **who should undergo pre-operative assessment** **when and where it should take place** **what is appropriate in terms of accurate record-keeping**		Tick	**& date**
2. Clinical thinking	Either write replies to this section or talk it through with assessor, who will initial each successful element **State the clinical problem exactly** **Clinical reasoning** 1. What was learnt through OBSERVATION? 2. Identify salient elements of HISTORY. 3. What were the reasons for INVESTGATIONS? 4. How have results been INTERPRETED? 5. Specify clinical conclusion accurately. 6. Identify risks and benefits of this. 7. How has this been shaped to the individual patient?		**Assessor's Initials**	
3. Actions	**Component elements** Interacts appropriately with patient Listens in focused way Asks appropriate and probing questions Can take informed consent & explain risks Can plan inter-operative management Can plan post-operative care Communicates appropriately with the multi-disciplinary team	**Self-assessment date & sig**	**Assessor date and sig**	

4. **Reflective overview**
What have you learnt that you will incorporate into everyday practice in future?
In what aspects of this do you feel you need further practice or assistance?

Do you feel competent to do the following in similar cases:
      1. engage successfully in these actions unsupervised?   YES / NO
      2. engage in this clinical thinking unsupervised?   YES / NO
      3. undertake pre-operative assessment unassisted   YES / NO

What extra help would assist to improve your competence in this skill?
This record has now been completed successfully **Supervisor signature:** …………………………………   **Date:** ……………………

It will be evident from this that we have required the context for the skill assessment to be documented; that we have provided more opportunity for learners to consider all the elements that influence and affect the performance of these skills, especially their thinking and knowing; and we have encouraged both written and spoken reflection.

We then developed a short course with educational goals (ten sessions of three hours each) to support the practical work, the recognition of the complexity of what underlies the skill, and the processes of reflection. (This has meant offering the SHOs involved some principles and processes for learning from practice more generally and they have reported that they are already using them whenever they think about their practice.)

As we write, this work is on-going. We refer to it here because it is currently giving us encouragement that there is a process for turning training into education, and because it offers the principles on which we worked to do so.

Equipped with the educational arguments, principles and processes, we can now turn to the detail of enacting these in surgical education.

Part two

Teaching, learning and assessing
in surgical settings

Introduction

'Learning to assess and reassess one's own competence and its limits, is a long and complex process, which becomes increasingly sophisticated as a doctor progresses through postgraduate education. Its reliability depends on access to good supervision...'

                            (Eraut and du Boulay, 2000, p. 4 of executive summary)

There is less time and there are fewer resources now than ever before for educating surgeons so that they progress along the pathway described thus by Eraut.

The second half of this book is dedicated to helping educators to enable learning surgeons to develop towards self-assessment as speedily, but also as rigorously, as possible. It is therefore addressed to all the key persons who facilitate the developing understanding of learning surgeons. It seeks to enable such educators to think reflectively and analytically about their *own* practice as well as that of their learners. It therefore looks in detail at how, through reflective discussion and writing, *knowledge, thought and action* can be analyzed, brought together, developed, extended and assessed, so that wise practice can be nurtured.

In all professions, the understanding of these matters is what underlies the serious and rigorous preparation of professionals of the future. Whether they are aware of it or not, how surgeon educators conceive of knowledge, thought and action and their inter-relationship (together with the more general relationship between theory and practice), inevitably influences all aspects of their teaching.

This is why we are arguing that cultivating a thinking surgeon involves focusing on the development of both the clinical thinking and the knowledge that underlie intelligent surgical practice in the clinical setting.

In the phrase 'intelligent surgical practice', we characterize intelligence more widely than as relating to mind alone. We believe that high quality surgeons, like every successful member of all professions, inevitably need to call upon their whole being in order to provide a sensible, sensitive and defensible service to their patients and clients. We therefore gloss the term 'intelligent' so as to recognize emotional intelligence and the multiple intelligences or frames of mind that Gardner has revealed, as seven ways of knowing the world (language; logical/mathematical analysis; spatial representation; musical thinking; the use of the body to solve problems or make things; an understanding of other individuals; and an understanding of ourselves). (See Gardner, 1993.)

In all professions, it is intelligent practice that underpins, and is manifested in, wise action. For health care professionals this depends upon specialist thinking, reasoning and knowing, which can only be fully learnt by taking real responsibility as a practising doctor or surgeon in the clinical setting, and which is far wider than that which it is possible to teach undergraduates.

It is the responsibility of educators at postgraduate level to enable inexperienced but working practitioners to come to grips with these matters.

In the education of surgeons, they must do so, of course, by using the realities of the working situation, where the particular context is crucial, problems are ill-structured and not easily formulated, the environment is uncertain, Trust requirements and resources can be inflexible, goals are shifting and competing, time is always pressing, and there are multiple versions of reality, because there are many people involved in the problem (both colleagues, the patient and the patient's supporters).

In this context, as Eraut points out: 'the central problem of postgraduate [medical] education is how best to combine work within a doctor's current competence, itself a source of learning, with the provision and use of learning opportunities to extend that competence' (Eraut and du Boulay, 2000, p.1 of executive summary).

Surgeon educators must therefore look to use examples from within the learner's current responsibilities, but also should seek wherever possible to stretch the learner into new examples and new areas of thought and action, which draw upon new knowledge, or require what is known to be re-structured and re-appraised. Good teachers challenge and support learners to reach towards that which is just within their grasp. This means that teachers must unpack the tacit thinking, understanding, knowing and being, that they have long been using but which lies invisible beneath their practice, so as to enable learners to see and explore it, and begin to make it their own through genuinely exploratory dialogue.

Bearing this in mind, Chapters 7 and 8 lead the reader through an exploration of clinical thinking of the kind that surgeons draw upon in their practice, and ways of teaching and assessing this. Chapter 9 turns to a consideration of the kinds of knowledge that underlie and underpin surgical practice, and Chapter 10 draws these together by focusing on the surgeon's main *raison d' être*, engagement in clinical and surgical processes and procedures, and the teaching and assessment of these. Finally, in Chapter 11, we offer some approaches to developing and extending both surgical and educational practice through practitioner research.

Chapter 7

Understanding and developing clinical thinking

Introduction: the importance of clinical thinking

Clinical thinking: a broad overview
    Introducing the key concepts
    The main components of clinical thinking
    Distinguishing between clinical reasoning and deliberation

Defining and exploring further the key concepts within clinical thinking
    Complex clinical problems
    How problem setting might be taught and learnt
    Clinical reasoning
    How clinical reasoning might be taught and learnt
    Personal professional judgement
    How such judgement might be taught and learnt
    Clinical solutions (options)
    How reaching a clinical solution might be taught and learnt
    Deliberation (or practical reasoning)
    How deliberation might be taught and learnt
    Practical wisdom
    How practical wisdom might be taught and learnt
    A professional judgement
    How reaching a professional judgement might be taught and learnt
    End notes

Education for clinical thinking: three pathways and their educational uses
    Example one (see Figure 7:3)
    The scenario of a new outpatient consultation
    Example two (see Figure 7:4)
    The scenario of new clinical thinking during treatment
    Example three (see Figure 7:5)
    A scenario of the wider issues of clinical practice
    The importance of revisiting decisions and thinking at all stages

End note

Introduction: the importance of clinical thinking

Specialist thinking is the very core of a professional's practice. It can link 'knowing' and 'being' to 'doing', and thus develop intelligent action. The essential question for all professionals is: 'what ought to be done, and how should and can we do it, given what we know of the situation in hand'? (see Golby and Parrott, 1999, p. 22). At the heart of any health care practitioner's conduct lie the reasoning used, the professional judgement exercised, and the clinical and professional conclusions reached, in respect of each specific patient. As before, we use the word 'conduct' here to signal that we are interested in not only the professional's visible behaviour, but also the motivations that drive it. These we see as shaped by the practitioner's underlying humanity and self-knowledge, and underpinned by moral and ethical sensitivity to the individual patient and particular context. We use the overall term 'clinical thinking' in this chapter to encompass the whole of these processes for doctors in the clinical setting.

Arriving at a sound professional decision in complex clinical situations is a key and unavoidable responsibility of the professional, and the exercise of such duty usually separates professionals from laymen. But fulfilling this responsibility is neither as easy, nor as scientific and objective, as it sounds. The contextual information, the patient narrative, the professional knowledge, and the scientific evidence which fuel the professional's thinking, are all inevitably incomplete, and/or require interpretation and sensitive reprocessing, and then have to be further customized to the individual patient case. Indeed, 'professional knowledge is essentially knowledge-in-action. It is often necessarily incomplete' (Golby and Parrott, 1999, p.22). There can be no 'cook-book' solutions here. As a classic text of evidence-based medicine noted, the clinician's individual judgements are always vital. It argues that:

> [because medicine] 'requires a bottom-up approach that integrates the best external evidence with individual clinical expertise and patient choice, it cannot result in slavish 'cook-book' approaches to individual patient care. External evidence can inform, but never replace, individual clinical expertise and it is this expertise that decides whether external evidence applies to the individual patient at all, and if so, how it should be integrated into a clinical decision.'
>
> (Sackett *et al*, 1997, p. 4)

For doctors generally, the reasoning and deliberation engaged in at the patient consultation stage, to frame the problem and reach a diagnosis, crucially set the course for all the following patient/professional encounters. During those later encounters, these same processes shape and reshape the professional's subsequent actions. Throughout patient care, doctors are accountable for their actions, and the decisions and reasoning which led to them. Further, given the litigious nature of our society in the 21st Century, these decision-making processes are also often the starting point for prosecution and defence, in cases where medical error is being investigated. The professional therefore needs to be able to be clear-thinking and articulate about them.

For surgeons in particular, the processes of clinical reasoning and decision-making are about whether and how to engage in surgical intervention for the individual patient, and how to manage that patient's treatment, after care and support. During their initial encounters with each patient, surgeons, unlike most other doctors, make and agree crucial decisions which are the gateway to serious and direct surgical action. This involves a licensed assault on a human being, from which there is often no turning back. During treatment and follow-up there will be many further occasions on which the surgeon will take the full responsibility for making overall sense of a problem, coming to a decision and acting - often speedily and in some cases without being able to consult the anaesthetised patient further. In the practice of a consultant surgeon these processes are complex, largely tacit, and are made fast and with practised fluency.

We would argue that inexperienced doctors or surgeons are often characterized by remarkable, but unfounded, certainty about clinical matters. Once in practice, they need as soon as possible to recognize the complexity of situations by learning these reasoning processes. Indeed, such processes need to be a central focus of the surgical curriculum. It seems to us that the more experienced clinicians become, the more they recognize complexity and uncertainty in practice and the need for the frequent exercise of professional judgement. The really safe practitioner may indeed be the one who always expects to exercise such judgement. The traditional phrase: 'It takes a surgeon not to operate!' reminds us that when all the apparently objective indications, (as identified during the clinical reasoning process), would lead the inexperienced surgeon to an unwise operative intervention, the careful deliberation of the senior surgeon often culminates in a more sound professional judgement *not* to intervene. Although clinical reasoning and professional judgement are clearly respected and valued in this kind of way within the senior surgical profession, they are rarely made explicit and examined, and their significance for surgical education is only now becoming recognized.

This is somewhat surprising, since those very surgical procedures - which the learning surgeon is motivated most urgently to acquire - cannot even be begun until the initial thinking and decision-making have been rigorously attended to, and certainly cannot be engaged in safely without sharp awareness of the moment by moment judgements which are part of surgical activity. Yet, until now, surgical procedures and their related pre-operative and post-operative processes, have been seen as the main core of surgical teaching, and learners have mostly been left to grasp the principles of sound clinical thinking and good judgement and to try to develop their facility in them, by osmosis. This often involves surgical teachers in acting as models. For example, they announce the clinical decision and leave learners to observe their visible actions, without making them privy to the whole of the thinking that underlies decision and action, (or perhaps not even being aware of much of it). Or it can lead educators to make explicit (or ask the learner to give a commentary about) only those elements of reasoning that are overt, or which can easily be articulated and described most straightforwardly. At worst this can unintentionally distort the vital process of clinical thinking in a number of obvious ways, and at best it does not do justice to the complexities of real surgical practice.

It is also the case that until recently the assessment of the learning surgeon's clinical reasoning, deliberative processes and professional judgement, have only been carried out implicitly within more general assessments of the learner's work in clinical settings. It has neither drawn on hard evidence of, nor generated any detailed records of, achievement in this area. This state of affairs has not promoted enduring confidence from the wider audience.

Neither does it match the growth of understanding of such matters (including assessment of them) in many of the other professions allied to medicine. And it will certainly not be sustainable in the face of increased government surveillance of surgery and surgical education in the 21st Century.

It therefore seems clear that for learning surgeons, these are crucial processes, in which they now need to be taught directly and assessed rigorously. All this sets a particular challenge for the surgical educator who must be able to surface, and make explicit and discuss the details of these hitherto tacit and taken-for-granted processes, who must find ways of enabling learners to understand and exercise them, and who then must encourage open ways of capturing and assessing them, so that achievement in them can be recorded and understood by new teachers and colleagues later in the young surgeon's career. This chapter offers support in respect of teaching and learning these matters. The following chapter takes up the details of assessment.

This chapter, therefore, provides an overview of the main processes within clinical thinking, followed by some key definitions and explorations of the major concepts which offer the vocabulary needed by surgical teacher and learner for considering the detail of their own practice. This first main section, which also offers ideas for teaching and learning these processes, is followed by a second, which offers some key examples of pathways leading to different kinds of clinical decisions.

Clinical thinking: a broad overview

Introducing the key concepts

There is considerable literature, across both medicine and a wide range of health care professions, which refers to a variety of ideas about what is involved in the clinical thinking which professionals engage in while making decisions about patient care. Many of the thinking processes, which lead to professional judgement, have in the last decade been widely explored and discussed within the health care professions (see especially: Fish and Coles, 1998; Higgs and Jones, 2002; Mattingly and Fleming, 1994; and the work of Benner in nursing). In medicine, statistical models to support decision-making, based mainly on Bayes theorem, have been in vogue with some since the 1960s (see White and Stancombe, 2003, pp. 9-13). Other authors have focused on illness scripts (Schmidt *et al*, 1992); and on pattern recognition (Patel and Groen, 1986). More recently, there have been wider approaches to medical decision-making in the work of Atkinson, (1995); Cox, (1999); Dowie and Elstein, (1988); Downie and Macnaughton, (2000); and White and Stancombe, (2003). The trend here has been towards drawing on science together with the humanities and arts to understand and illuminate the thinking processes involved. For example, the collection edited by Dowie and Elstein offers chapters on everything from mathematical models to intuitive thinking, while Atkinson stresses the significance of talk in the processes leading to judgement, and the importance of analyzing and interpreting it. The two most recent texts listed above explicitly refer to the role of science and the arts in clinical decision-making.

Throughout this literature various terms are given to clinical thinking. These include: clinical reasoning; clinical decision-making, medical decision-making and medical reasoning. There is as yet no agreement about them, either within or across professions. There is a broad consensus, however, that the term 'clinical reasoning', refers to a logical thought process of hypothetico-deductive reasoning, of pattern recognition, or of 'forward or backward (inductive and deductive) thinking' (see especially: Higgs and Jones, 2002; Thompson and Dowding, 2002; and White and Stancombe, 2003). The term 'professional judgement' is also frequently used by many writers, but in our view most do not make a clear enough distinction between it and clinical reasoning. We note with interest that Cox, (1999), like us, uses clinical thinking as the term to encompass the entire process.

Aware that these were the issues emerging from the literature, we chose to try to disentangle these concepts and identify the key ones, by analyzing the practices of surgeons in the clinical setting. We did so by asking them to capture elements of their clinical work and to explore these with us in detail. By these means we came to tease apart clinical reasoning from deliberation, as two very different thinking processes, which result in two different kinds of decisions about practice, and which need each other, but which, initially at least, can usefully be understood, taught and assessed, separately.

The main components of clinical thinking

In Figure 7:1 on page 137, we show the key components of clinical thinking, and their basic linear relationship. We show such thinking as beginning with a *complex clinical problem* (within the context of patient care). We use the word 'complex' here, because we believe that the term 'medical or surgical decision' best encompasses the relatively simple response to answers to closed questions about fairly uncomplicated clinical activities (shall I put up a drip here? shall I order a CT scan? shall I prescribe drug X or Y?). Here, only the most simple pros and cons need to be considered before a clear-cut decision, which is quickly self-validating, is made. Medical/surgical decisions are often overlooked by expert surgeons, who make them tacitly and fast, as part of their knowledge-in-action in a given situation. Learners may need to rehearse the pros and cons aloud and check out their appropriateness and that of the decision reached, but this can be done quite thoroughly through brief discussion at the time.

By contrast, the complex clinical problem (which may be a patient's problem or about an aspect of Trust policy) is construed by the surgeon, alone or in consultation with patients and colleagues, as part of the clinical thinking process. Such *case formulation* draws upon the surgeon's (patients' and colleagues') values, beliefs and experience. Formulation of the problem then triggers the need for *clinical reasoning*. This seeks, through neutral logic and scientific knowledge, which are not contextualized to the patient, to identify and explore those elements and actions that will be significant in the resolution of the problem. This in turn leads to an objectified and generalized *clinical conclusion or conclusions* about what is the right thing to do generally in cases such as this.

Doctors then need to situate this generalized logic, and adapt this neutral clinical solution, to the needs of the specific individual patient within the particular clinical context. They do so by engaging in *deliberation*, which weighs, prioritizes and responds to the context-specific demands and pressures. These emanate from: the patient's needs; the clinician's views, vision, abilities, knowledge; and the requirements and possibilities of the particular Trust. *Practical wisdom* (or what Aristotle calls *phronesis*) then helps the practitioner to focus on and understand the particular ethical dimensions and moral situation of this individual patient. This thinking process leads to *a professional judgement*, which is a decision about the best action to be taken in this particular patient's case. It is the end result of the whole process of clinical thinking. Where practical wisdom has been harnessed to consider the moral and ethical issues, the resulting activity can be referred to as *wise action* or what Aristotle calls *praxis* (see Carr, 1995, p. 71). Each stage, together with its associated decision-making, must of course be kept under frequent review.

However, there is one more vital element. Since medicine is an imperfect science, complications can arise at all points in its practice. See Gawande, (2001), for surgical examples. He makes the point that:

'Professionals are routinely faced with having to decide which diagnosis or whose version or account of the [patient's] troubles they find most convincing and/or morally robust.'

(Gawande, 2001, p. ix)

He also says that medicine is:

'... an enterprise of constantly changing knowledge, uncertain information, fallible individuals, ... There is science in what we do, yes, but also habit, intuition, and sometimes plain old guessing. The gap between what we know and what we aim for persists. And this gap complicates everything we do.'

(Gawande, 2001, p. 7)

Although they are presented in simple terms in Figure 7:1, therefore, none of the thinking processes endemic to clinical reasoning and deliberation is actually simple. Indeed, there is a need in each of them, at all points, to identify the salient features involved, to weigh the significance of various elements, and to interpret the meaning of even the most scientific of evidence. This even includes the formulation of the complex clinical problem in itself. Further, all human situations are constantly evolving, and there is always a need for professionals to continue to respond to developments and to refine or reconsider their conclusions. In response, the professional practitioner's vital capacity to exercise *personal professional judgement* comes into play at all points, from formulating the complex clinical problem to reaching the final professional judgement. It enables the surgeon to deal with complexity, with competing demands, and with the ambiguities which all too often arise in evolving human interaction. Unlike the (public) professional judgement or decision, referred to above, which is the end product of the whole process of clinical thinking, this personal professional judgement is an ability, which is exercised, to weigh up competing elements, ideas, and actions. It involves adjudicating between conflicting priorities, where soundness of common sense and steadiness of focus are essential. Figure 7:1 therefore shows that at the core of clinical thinking lies the personal professional judgement of the clinician.

We believe that these key elements and their basic relationship as mapped in Figure 7:1, are the foundation of any kind of clinical thinking which begins with the formulation of a complex problem and ends with the start of, or plan for, wise action, although of course some elements

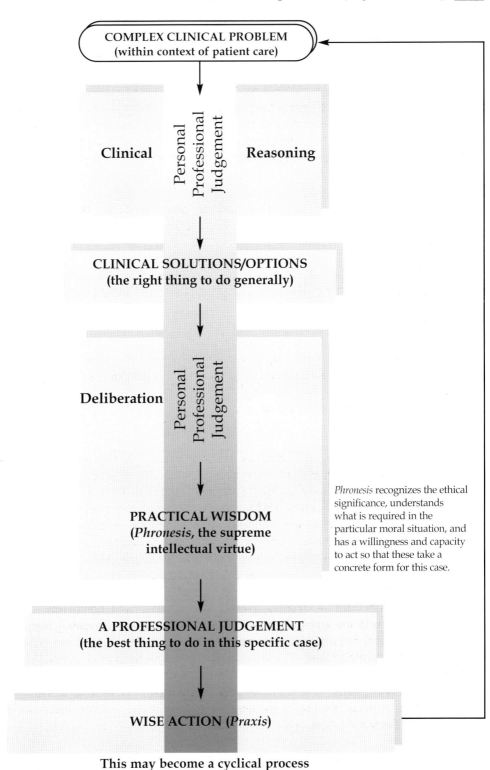

COMPLEX CLINICAL PROBLEM
(within context of patient care)

Clinical   Personal Professional Judgement   Reasoning

CLINICAL SOLUTIONS/OPTIONS
(the right thing to do generally)

Deliberation   Personal Professional Judgement

PRACTICAL WISDOM
(*Phronesis*, the supreme intellectual virtue)

Phronesis recognizes the ethical significance, understands what is required in the particular moral situation, and has a willingness and capacity to act so that these take a concrete form for this case.

A PROFESSIONAL JUDGEMENT
(the best thing to do in this specific case)

WISE ACTION (*Praxis*)

This may become a cyclical process

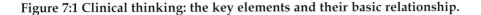

Figure 7:1 Clinical thinking: the key elements and their basic relationship.

will be present in greater or lesser degrees depending on the nature of the problem. Thus, this general pathway can be used to explore such thinking, whether it is focused on the process that leads from the first outpatient consultation to an agreed treatment plan, is concerned with the thinking that leads to wise action within the treatment itself, or is looking for the resolution of wider clinical issues.

Distinguishing between clinical reasoning and deliberation

The two main forms of reasoning within clinical thinking (clinical reasoning on the one hand and deliberation, or practical reasoning on the other), are greatly contrasting in nature, as follows.

Clinical reasoning

In its simplest and purest form, clinical reasoning construes the complex clinical problem as a technical one. It then operates through a formula to solve a clinical problem (comes to a clinical conclusion) by using a straightforward set of rules, and assumes that what counts as evidence would be agreed by everyone.

A key example of clinical reasoning (generally referred to as 'diagnostic reasoning') involves coming to a working diagnosis. From this viewpoint, clinical reasoning can be seen as a bio-medical process, which distinguishes the disease from the patient, and regards the problem as to do with malfunctioning parts of the patient. It is a technical problem, requiring technical competence from the practitioner. It is based on logic and order, collects predictable categories of evidence, and uses a formulaic approach to reach a clinical decision. It claims a scientific basis, and stems from a world view that sees facts as objective, precise, and absolute, and truth as out there, waiting to be discovered. It assumes that scientific theory can be directly translated into practice. It is deliberately devoid of moral and ethical concern.

Clinical reasoning (sometimes without this term being attached to it) is taught in this simple form at medical school. Indeed, we note in passing, at this stage, that traditionally this has been all that was taught at medical school. The processes of personal judgement at its core, (together with the processes of deliberation, the exercise of practical wisdom and the making of a final professional judgement), can only be learnt at postgraduate level by a doctor who takes professional responsibility in the clinical setting. Thus, newly qualified doctors are usually unaware that there is any more to clinical thinking than the simple version of clinical reasoning.

But, when 'the simplicities of science come up against the complexities of individual lives' (Gawande, 2001, p. 8), personal professional judgement has to be exercised and other important forms of clinical reasoning in response to a complex clinical problem are needed. For example, even in the most technical of patient cases, investigations must be selected, evidence must be interpreted and explanations found for it, and judgements must be made about when enough evidence is at hand. This may well require other versions of clinical reasoning beyond the traditional diagnostic/scientific reasoning with its hypothetico-deductive base. These are, narrative reasoning, and interactive reasoning. (We look at these in more detail in the next section). At postgraduate level, then, clinical reasoning takes on a more complex form and is illuminated at various points by personal/professional judgement. Nonetheless, it still follows a logical order, still sees the problem and its solution in broadly scientific terms, and thus can fairly readily be made overt by surgeon educators and shared with and developed in their learners. It can then be assessed orally and in writing.

Deliberation

By contrast, deliberation always recognizes the complexity at the core of clinical thinking, and sees clinical problems as humane problems, which are inevitably characterized by messiness and uncertainty, and which require an echoing human response from the practitioner. Deliberation holds as an open question what would count as evidence in respect of its arguments. It thus needs to draw on professionals' personal judgement processes, and practical wisdom, to produce a professional decision, which in turn leads to a wise action. Young doctors who have not recognized deliberation as a significant process of clinical thinking during medical school are often shocked to discover its central importance in medical practice.

A key example of deliberation is the process which turns a working diagnosis into a treatment plan for a particular patient, and which has been agreed by that patient and others involved. Deliberation, then, is grounded in the professional's humanity and concerned with the patient's social being in the world. It calls upon imagination and compassion in the practitioner to help him/her understand how the patient is seeing and feeling and thus interpret more sensitively what they want and need. It draws on knowledge of science and life, sensitivity to language, understanding of social interaction, and recognition of what is involved at a human level in constructing a history. Further, it admits the existence of emotional elements in the patient's story and the practitioner's response. It sees disease as a breakdown of the patient's social world, and crucially recognizes that the meaning of any situation is likely to be construed differently by each of the different people involved in it. (That is, it believes both in the social construction of knowledge and in multiple versions of reality).

Deliberation draws on the artistry of the practitioner. That is, it involves recognizing the unique nature of the situation, engaging in a dialogue with that situation, and being ready to go beyond the rules (see Schön, 1987, p. 22). It is based on pragmatic and practical reasoning in which human and equally competing priorities vie for attention, in an order which has to arise from the particulars of the problem and which will therefore be different for different patients. It thus eschews formulae for thinking, using instead an investigative approach to unearthing all the pertinent elements and a reflective and critical approach to prioritizing and weighing them up. It is based on a view of the world as complex, ambiguous, and uncertain. It works from practice to theory. Typically, it involves the clinician in appreciating patients' experiences of illness such as their feelings and fears about being ill; their ideas about what is wrong with them and the basis of those ideas; the impact of the problem on their lives; their expectations about what should be done; and their sense of control or powerlessness in relation to their situation (see Higgs, Jones, Edwards, *et al*, 2004, p 190). Practical wisdom is what enables the practitioner to focus on and be sensitive to the moral and ethical dimensions involved.

Deliberation has the practitioner's personal professional judgement at its heart and is more difficult to articulate. Indeed, professional artistry 'does not depend on our being able to describe what we know how to do or even to entertain in conscious thought the knowledge our actions reveal' (Schön, 1987, p. 22). Thus, 'the knowledge involved in our knowledgeable actions is *tacit*, and difficult to bring to the surface' (Fish, 1998, p. 55). Surgeon educators will need to unearth this tacit knowledge in order to share it with the learner, and foster the development of it in the learner. It can then be assessed through the learner's narrative of ideas, events, thinking, doing, knowing and feeling that fed into the judgement reached (see also Chapter 9).

We offer these ideas (summarized in Figure 7:2), to enable surgical teachers and learners to begin to explore the ways of thinking endemic to each of these processes.

We wish to make it clear, however, that this model (like all diagrams) simplifies and reduces real-life complexities. For example, we do not see these processes as solitary activities leading to decisions by lone professionals. Nor do we see them as necessarily happening within a short and simple linear time scale. We also recognize with White and Stancombe that 'case formulations often remain unarticulated in encounters with patients ... and may not exist as single events produced spontaneously on discrete occasions ... [but] emerge gradually over time and through conversation with colleagues.' (White and Stancombe, 2003, p.14). We also recognize with Atkinson that the clinical setting involves both single-professional and multi-professional teams, and is like all other organizational settings where 'decision-making itself is a collective organizational activity ... [where decisions are] subject to debate, negotiation and revision, based on talk within and between groups or teams of practitioners [and where] the silent inner dialogue of single-handed decision-making ... is by no means the whole story,' (Atkinson, 1995, p. 52). Further, we acknowledge that in human interaction, one person's way of making meaning out of a situation can never precisely match another's.

Defining and exploring further the key concepts within clinical thinking

We can now offer the following definitions and explorations of the main elements in clinical thinking. We do so in order that surgical teachers and learners will have a stable and shared language in which to talk together and begin to record the solid (written) evidence of the learner's achievements in these areas. These definitions are broadly consonant with those in the current literature, and are (we believe) particular to the needs of surgeons. Their standardized use, in our view, will enhance for surgeons the processes of teaching, learning and assessment in the clinical setting. Under each heading we offer a definition, an exploration (with example or examples where relevant), and a comment on how these matters can be taught and learnt (together in some cases, with action points for teacher and learner).

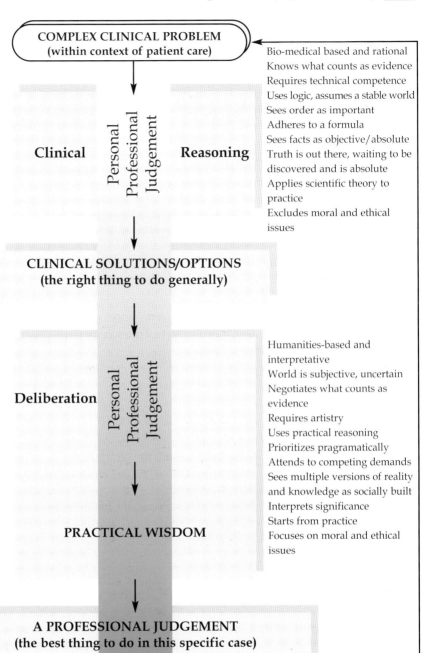

Framing the problem involves: processing narratives and using judgement and diagnostic reasoning at first, and then later other reasoning processes.

Once clinical reasoning is seen to demand interpretation and prioritization, then personal professional judgement can signal and attend to the complexities that underlie this scientific approach. Then clinical reasoning turns to narrative and other forms of reasoning.

Deliberative processes include:

recognizing all the relevant elements;
accepting the humane nature of the problem;
contextualizing;
seeing multiple views;
interpreting;
prioritizing;
attributing significance.

It draws on:
science, language, social interaction, history, emotion and practical wisdom.

Practical wisdom enlightens deliberation by linking it to the particular moral context.

COMPLEX CLINICAL PROBLEM
(within context of patient care)

Bio-medical based and rational
Knows what counts as evidence
Requires technical competence
Uses logic, assumes a stable world
Sees order as important
Adheres to a formula
Sees facts as objective/absolute
Truth is out there, waiting to be discovered and is absolute
Applies scientific theory to practice
Excludes moral and ethical issues

Clinical Personal Professional Judgement **Reasoning**

CLINICAL SOLUTIONS/OPTIONS
(the right thing to do generally)

Deliberation Personal Professional Judgement

Humanities-based and interpretative
World is subjective, uncertain
Negotiates what counts as evidence
Requires artistry
Uses practical reasoning
Prioritizes pragramatically
Attends to competing demands
Sees multiple versions of reality and knowledge as socially built
Interprets significance
Starts from practice
Focuses on moral and ethical issues

PRACTICAL WISDOM

A PROFESSIONAL JUDGEMENT
(the best thing to do in this specific case)

WISE ACTION

This may become a cyclical process

Figure 7:2 Clinical thinking: a broad overview.

Complex clinical problems

Definition

We have shown that complex clinical problems can be defined in contrast to simple ones, which are expressed in a closed question. We can define complex clinical problems as open questions about complex clinical matters (which focus either directly on agreeing the patient's treatment plan, or on the patient's treatment processes), or more broadly on issues related to the care of patients while in the Trust.

Exploration

Complex clinical problems, however, do not spring out of the air fully formed. They are inside the process of clinical thinking. How complex clinical problems are construed by the clinician is highly significant and will determine the nature of the rest of the clinical thinking. Framing the complex clinical problem is known as problem setting or case formulation, (and is often given less attention than problem solving). Problem setting is 'the process by which we define the decision to be made, the ends to be achieved, and the means which may be chosen' to achieve such ends (Schön, 1987, pp. 65-66).

Clinical problems are most likely to be seen by surgeons as purely technical problems, as technical problems with humane dimensions, or as humane problems with technical dimensions. There may, of course, be some clinical problems that are purely technical, but most will have human connotations. It should be noted, however, that such characterization is not simply endemic to the nature of the problem, but rather the problem has been assigned a character by the surgeon. How problems are framed will depend on the surgeon's view of the world and his/her personal values, priorities, beliefs, theories and assumptions. This is also affected by those lenses brought habitually by the surgeon to viewing clinical problems (and the rest of his/her world). As Brookfield, 2002 p. 65, shows, it should be remembered that even the basic process of observation of the patient within diagnostic reasoning can be coloured by the lenses through which we look. He lists the key lenses as: those which are shaped by the clinician's own autobiography; those in which the clinician takes on the eyes of the patient; and those borrowed from other colleagues' life-knowledge and experience.

Some surgeons inhabit what Schön, (1987), called the 'hard high ground' of professional certainty, and may routinely construe clinical problems as technical or mainly technical, or may simply see their technical nature as 'given'. (Though this of course may be because they have never overtly questioned their approach to problem setting.) Problems thus characterized are seen as needing only basic verification before leading to investigation by the specialist. In such cases, the pure form of clinical diagnostic reasoning will be seen as appropriate and even sufficient to their solution, and will provide a clinical conclusion that is satisfyingly scientific and thus dependable in leading to a straightforward decision to act.

For others, however, clinical problems are more likely to be seen as inhabiting the 'swampy lowlands' or 'indeterminate zones' of practice (see Schön, 1987). For these surgeons, the complex clinical problem is not *a given*, which comes to the clinician fully fledged. Rather, it is construed by the surgeon from a mixture of (for example), prior diagnoses which may themselves be in conflict (that of the patient not in agreement with that of the referring GP, for example); the patient's narrative; puzzling and complicated signs and symptoms; and observable evidence, examinations and tests. All this is seen as needing to be understood within the context of each specific patient's case, the individual Trust's expectations and requirements, and the practitioner's own knowledge and practical experience. In such cases, the problem is likely to be seen as multi-dimensional, needing various forms of clinical reasoning (narrative reasoning, etc.) and professional judgement, and appealing for its validity to practical experience, common sense, professional status, professional judgement and collegiate agreement.

How problem setting might be taught and learnt

Problem setting can be (and needs to be) directly taught and learnt through professional conversations between the surgeon educator and the learning surgeon, in which these ideas are firstly critiqued *as ideas*, and then used to critique real practice. This cannot begin, however, until the teacher has prepared for it, by being able to unearth and critique his/her own tacit knowledge of, and pre-suppositions and assumptions about, this process.

Clinical reasoning

Definition

In common with much of the literature, we use the term clinical reasoning to characterize the gamut of clinical decision-making processes in which surgeons engage. By clinical reasoning we mean those broadly logical, straightforwardly ordered, (and to some extent formulaic) thinking and acting processes in clinical practice which lead a clinician who has formulated a complex clinical problem to come to a clinical conclusion about it. There are a number of forms of clinical reasoning.

The process appears at first to involve technical reasoning, relying on calculations to determine a course of action, focusing on utility and probability and reducing the clinical world to 'emotionless space for the administration of clinical calculus' (White and Stancombe, 2003, p. 14). This is a pure form of diagnostic reasoning. However, as we have seen, most complex clinical problems have strong human dimensions, which demand rather more than a scientific response, and call on other versions of clinical reasoning. Indeed, in the literature of the wider health care professions, there are listed many forms of clinical reasoning which attend to the human complexities arising for both the patient and the clinician. We explore these below.

Exploration

At its simplest the key basic processes of clinical reasoning as used in diagnosis are history taking, physical examination, and investigation. When the results of these are brought up to the propositional medical knowledge (text book information and research knowledge), a diagnosis can be formulated by means of a logic which discounts each of a range of possibilities, until the field is narrowed to a close fit between evidence and its unequivocal meaning. This process, known as differential diagnosis, relies on hypothetico-deductive reasoning and is founded on the work of Karl Popper (and ideas about proof by refutation). The virtues of this are considered to be that the thinking involved is scientific and therefore objective (in that it is uncomplicated by the specifics of the case, and relies on the notion that truth is universal). We fully accept of course, that, technology and technical thinking are an indispensable bedrock in biomedicine. However, as we have shown, much medicine is found to be an imperfect science, in which personal judgement plays an inevitable and vital part of this process. Once this is recognized, then additional forms of clinical reasoning become important.

Kinds of reasoning useful for surgeons in the clinical reasoning stage of clinical thinking

The following provides a list of forms of clinical reasoning which we have adapted from our own investigations of surgical practice and the work of Higgs and of Cox (see Higgs, 2003, p. 150; Higgs, Jones, Edwards, *et al*, 2004, p. 183; and Cox, 1999.) We have divided the whole list as found in Higgs' work, between clinical reasoning and deliberation, although she does not make these distinctions. We would point out that many of the four forms of reasoning listed by us within clinical reasoning are automatically drawn on to respond to the human elements of a patient case, as part of diagnostic reasoning. They come under the heading of reasoning because all have a logic and order intrinsic to them, which they bring to shape the surgeon's thinking, and they are about understanding the complex clinical problem. They are as follows:

1. **Hypothetico-deductive reasoning** (generation of hypotheses based on clinical data and knowledge, and testing these hypotheses through further enquiry in order to make a clinical decision, as shown in Figure 7:1).

2. **Diagnostic reasoning** (the reasoning that starts with a complex clinical problem and proceeds to a clinical conclusion, as shown in the top half of Figure 7:2). In real practice it involves far more than pure science and logic.

3. **Interactive reasoning** (this occurs when dialogue with colleagues and the multi-disciplinary team is used deliberately to enhance or facilitate the clinical thinking process). This would be expected, to a greater or lesser extent, to be a part of all clinical thinking engaged in by the learning surgeon.

4. **Narrative reasoning** (involves the use of telling and listening to stories in order to understand a clinical problem more deeply). Examples would include the importance, in diagnosis, of the patient's story; or, during post-operative care, of the patient's supporters' stories; or perhaps, in seeking to change Trust policy, of the importance of tracing that policy's history through the stories of various interested parties. In all cases, narrative reasoning is about hearing, interpreting and re-telling stories. These narratives recapitulate and attend to temporal sequence, contextualize and offer the antecedents and consequences of events, attribute cause and effect, construct blameworthiness and credit-worthiness, and are often moral tales (see White and Stancombe, 2003, p. 20). Attention to the subtleties and colour of words is important here in piecing together how reality is seen and understood by the talker.

We list later in this chapter, six other narrative forms which are currently offered by Higgs as part of clinical reasoning but which we believe are versions of deliberation.

Higgs presents all these reasoning processes as having three core elements at their heart (see Higgs, Jones, Edwards, *et al*, 2004, p. 184). These are reflective enquiry, a strong discipline-specific multi-dimensional knowledge base, and metacognition. This last element refers to knowledge of the thinking processes themselves, together with the self-reflective awareness that allows clinicians to monitor the quality of information obtained, evaluate the limitations of their knowledge and thinking, and detect unexpected findings, like for example clinical data which do not fit the emerging clinical pattern (see Higgs, Jones, Edwards, *et al*, 2004, p. 196). We find this a useful summary.

How clinical reasoning might be taught and learnt

The basic processes of clinical reasoning are presented and learnt in medical school with the emphasis on their logic and rigour, as essential to ensuring the meticulous exploration of the patient's problem. The learning surgeon soon comes to discover that their apparently simple and scientific/logical neutrality and accuracy hides a great deal of ambiguity, that the salient facts are not always easy to disentangle from the peripheral ones, and that interpretation happens and personal judgement is needed, at all stages. They learn too that many patients give 'poor histories, cover up symptoms, seek to hide information that they think might expose them to blame or ridicule, have undiscovered ailments or have more than one disease at a time' (White and Stancombe, 2003, p. 12). They quickly discover that more than one hypothesis may be true at the same time, and that in the dialogue between the patient and the surgeon 'there is ample room for misunderstanding, incomplete versions and false trails' (White and Stancombe, 2003, p.6).

Learning surgeons further discover that their seniors cut many corners by relying on pattern recognition, or on inductive reasoning, combined with intuitive sensing of the salient features based on accumulated experience. Such abridged strategies, used by senior clinicians in the efficient pursuit of a clinical conclusion or final diagnosis, have been well documented (Glass,

1996; Kassirer and Kopelman, 1991; Newble and Cannon, 1994; Ridderikhoff, 1991; and Rimoldi, 1988). These 'typically establish an early context for continuing investigation and management by invoking one or more initial diagnoses, often arrived at by the recognition of a familiar set of data from a background of extensive knowledge of clinical features and prevelance of disease.' (Sefton, Gordon and Field, 2002, p. 188). Such expertise, of course, makes it difficult for surgical teachers in any given case to be aware of and make overt their thinking, so that its processes can be unpicked. It can lead the learner to be unaware of what really drives the clinical decision-making in more experienced colleagues. Worse, it often leaves the inexperienced learning surgeon 'caught between the admonition to be thorough and systematic in gathering and presenting clinical data, on the one hand, and pressure to reach efficient but appropriate diagnostic endpoints, on the other' (Sefton, Gordon and Field, 2002, p. 188).

Action points

We offer the following processes, ordered deliberately, to assist surgical teachers and learners, in working together, to explore in detailed discussion the process of clinical reasoning (in all its possible forms).

1. Begin by working together to understand and critique clinical reasoning, in its abstract form (as presented in Figure 7:2 and the elaboration in this section). Only by talking together and listening carefully can each party be sure that they have established a shared understanding of these processes.

2. The surgeon educator needs to unearth his/her tacit knowledge of these processes in relation to key examples of his/her own practice, drawn from three areas: processes leading to patients' treatment plans; those leading to patients' treatment processes; and, more broadly, those aimed at refining policies related to the care of patients while in the Trust. These real examples need to be used to critique the abstract ideas presented above, and the abstract ideas to understand and critique the real practice.

3. The surgeon educator then needs to share these examples of practice with the learning surgeon and encourage him/her to offer a commentary on them.

4. The learning surgeon also needs to be engaged in talking through the process in relation to a current patient case, during or at the end of the patient consultation stage and then during the treatment stage. Both teacher and learner can consider how far the details offered above enlighten the process.

5. The learning surgeon needs to practise clinical reasoning in relation to a range of current patients at both consultation and treatment stage.

6. At least one such case from consultation and from treatment need to be written up by the learning surgeon as a brief narrative, punctured by bracketed comments which

identify the parts of the process and then critiqued in bullet points (see, for example pages 172-173).

7.   The learning surgeon needs to be set a small project in which s/he outlines the clinical reasoning s/he would present to a policy group in seeking to refine or change Trust policy about some aspect of patient care.

Personal professional judgement

Definition

The surgeon's personal professional judgement is a capacity to be exercised. It should run throughout the whole of clinical thinking, influencing the construing of the complex clinical problem and then each of the subsequent processes used, together with their associated decisions. It refers to the ability of the professional to see beyond the technicalities of a situation and to recognize the need for wider forms of clinical reasoning or deliberation. It enables the professional: to see the salient features of a problem as needing interpretation; to regard the various elements that impinge upon it and its resolution as needing re-prioritizing; and to recognize the need to weigh the relative importance of each of them in respect of the case in hand and its particular context.

Exploration

Personal professional judgement harnesses common sense and the understanding gained through experience, in order to construe the case in hand as a humane (as well as a technical) problem. It might, for example, during clinical reasoning cause the surgeon to recognize and take account of the fact that there is no one absolute way of interpreting particular evidence, that the patient's story is only one way of making meaning out of a situation of complex meanings which are culturally determined, or that some elements of a case history need to be re-visited. During the deliberation process, it will be called on at all the moments when adjudication has to take place between competing priorities, to resolve ambiguities, or to assign relative significance to several elements.

How such judgement might be taught and learnt

The soundness of the learning surgeon's personal professional judgement can be elucidated from and assessed via a personal narrative aimed at demonstrating why personal judgement was needed in this case, and its role within the reasoning process. It is also possible to analyze the relevance and intelligence of the clinical processes utilized and decisions made in the name of professional judgement. We offer in the following chapter a detailed table to support the assessment of this (see pages 182-183).

Clinical solutions (options)

Definition

At its simplest, this is the medical or even scientific and technical end result (decision) of clinical reasoning. It is the culmination of the scientific investigation of the evidence collected. It is a generalized conclusion, in that it is generally the right thing to do in cases of this kind. It can be a technical resolution to a problem which is construed as technical, or it can be a conclusion about clinical problems which have been explored by a variety of forms of clinical reasoning.

Exploration

In relation to the initial consultations with a new patient, for example, the clinical conclusion can be a neutral and unequivocal diagnosis of what is wrong with them, and what to do about it, based on the evidence collected from that patient's history, physical examination and investigations. It can provide the clinician with a clear-cut way forward. That is, it provides a view about the given symptoms and the right way to treat them, based on knowledge built up from past patterns. At best such a clinical conclusion is an important starting point (a working diagnosis) for discussion with the patient, which will shape the agreed treatment plan. At worst it provides an unquestioned and unequivocal basis for action, which is more or less imposed upon the individual patient. When that is the case, it conflates the notion of what should be done (generally in cases like this), with what will be done (in this case), as if they were one and the same, and as if there were no other issues to be taken account of.

A clinical conclusion (or clinical judgement) however, 'is not and can never be Euclidian geometry'. Rather, as we have shown above, it is characterized by 'shifting formulations, carrying varying degrees of confidence' (White and Stancombe, 2003, p. 4). Under this view, the clinical conclusion (which may be the result of clinical reasoning focused on the patient consultation; on the treatment processes; or on a Trust's policy issue) represents the best approximation to a logical conclusion as is possible.

How reaching a clinical solution might be taught and learnt

The quality and appropriateness of the clinical conclusion, drawn as a result of clinical reasoning, can easily be made overt and discussed between surgeon educator and learning surgeon, through oral and written reflection. Paradoxically, the clinical conclusion reached by a learning surgeon who has engaged in the processes of professional judgement ought to be more tentative and more provisional than that reached by a medical student. Indeed, in postgraduate practice (unlike in medical school), clinical reasoning and clinical decision-making should be considered *critically*, in terms of the interpretative elements within it, and within a given context for an individual patient. We elaborate on the assessment of this in the following chapter.

Deliberation (or practical reasoning)

Definition

Deliberation is a process of thinking that focuses on the problematic and contestable issues endemic to practising as a professional. As Golby and Parrott, (1999), p. 24, point out, professionals 'have to [learn to] make contextualized judgements in the light of both local circumstances and the guiding principles of the practice'. Such reasoning is about deciding between competing and even conflicting moral ideals. (Sometimes all that is possible is respect for one value at the expense of another of equal weight.) In such a situation, it is impossible to resort to technical reasoning, which relies on calculations to determine what course of action to take.

Exploration

Deliberation (or practical reasoning) occurs when there are competing medical/surgical ways forward in coming to, and acting upon, a clinical decision. This involves coming to a final professional judgement by weighing up, in the context of the individual patient's case, the following: the clinical conclusion; the guiding principles of good practice; the specifics of the patient's views and cultural context; the competing demands of the given clinical/Trust setting; the professional practitioner's own values and abilities; and the views of other professional colleagues in the medical/surgical team. Such a weighing of the significance and salience of these matters means that personal judgement is also a necessary part of this process.

Deliberation about practice then is not a method for determining how to do something, but for deciding what ought to be done *in this case*, and where the outcomes of practice cannot be pre-specified. It must try to ascertain the relevant facts about the specific case and generate alternative solutions. It must make every effort to trace the branching pathways of consequences which may flow from each alternative. It must weigh alternatives and their costs and consequences against one another and choose not the right alternative, for there is no such thing as the right decision in respect of a general case, but only the best one in this case.

The process of deliberation interprets the messy and the inexact. It does not purport to treat this neutrally, analytically and objectively. It does not celebrate logic. So, the correctness of its ultimate professional judgement cannot be proved, but it can be validated by the opinions of others, and by subsequent events. Such a judgement is not reached by the exercise of deliberation alone. Indeed, it is possible to engage in deliberation as if it too were a mere technical process, of purely academic interest. What crucially prevents this from happening is the possession and exercising of practical wisdom. As Carr points out: 'Without practical wisdom, deliberation degenerates into an intellectual exercise and 'good practice' becomes indistinguishable from instrumental cleverness' (Carr, 1995, p. 71).

Several of the forms of thinking listed by Higgs, (2003), and Higgs, Jones, Edwards *et al*, (2004), we would see as part of deliberation (which she does not discuss as such). They are as follows.

Predictive reasoning

This refers to estimating the patient's likely responses to treatment and likely outcomes of management, based on information obtained through interview during the deliberative stage.

Creative/intuitive reasoning

This occurs when fresh approaches to a problem are called for, or when mismatches between elements under consideration are recognized because there is a sense that things do not fit.

Collaborative reasoning

This refers to shared decision-making with the patient, in which learning surgeons would expect to engage during the deliberative stage.

Teaching as reasoning

'This occurs when practitioners consciously use advice, instruction and guidance for the purpose of promoting change in the patient's understanding, feelings and behaviour' (see Higgs, 2003, p. 150).

Pragmatic reasoning

This we would call deliberation.

Ethical and moral reasoning

Following Aristotle, we prefer to call this practical wisdom.

How deliberation might be taught and learnt

Action points

As with clinical reasoning, it is useful to begin by working together to understand and critique deliberation, in its abstract form, and for the surgeon educator to unearth his/her tacit knowledge of deliberation in relation to key examples of his/her own practice: in coming to formulate patients' treatment plans; in patients' treatment processes; and, more broadly, in refining policies related to the care of patients while in the Trust. Here, again, theory needs to be used to critique practice and vice versa. The following processes then need to be engaged in.

1. The surgeon educator needs to share personal examples of deliberation with the learning surgeon and encourage him/her to identify the relevant pressures and demands bearing on the judgement to be made, and to map as far as possible the pathways which have led to the various adjudications.

2. The learning surgeon also needs to be engaged in talking through these processes in relation to a current patient case, and to practise deliberation in relation to a range of current patients at both consultation and treatment stage.

3. At least one entire mapping of deliberation in an example from presentation to treatment plan, and in a second example during treatment itself, needs to be written up by the learning surgeon. This should be a brief narrative, punctured by bracketed comments which identify the parts of the process and then critiqued in bullet points.

4. The learning surgeon needs to extend, with reference to deliberation, the small project associated with clinical reasoning in relation to refining or changing Trust policy about some aspect of patient care (as suggested above, p. 147).

Practical wisdom

Definition

This for Aristotle is the supreme intellectual virtue, and is about 'knowing which general ethical principles to apply in a particular situation' (Carr, 1995, p. 71). The doctor or surgeon who possesses practical wisdom is the professional who 'sees the particularities of the practical situation in the light of their ethical significance and acts consistently on this basis', to achieve the greatest good for the particular patient.

Exploration

The exercise of practical wisdom is made manifest in a practitioner who has:

'a knowledge of what is required in a particular moral situation and a willingness to act so that this knowledge can take concrete form. It is a comprehensive moral capacity which combines practical knowledge of the good with sound judgement about what, in a particular situation, would constitute an appropriate expression of this 'good'.'

(Carr, 1995, p. 71).

For example, having determined by deliberation what is the best way of providing quality care in this disease in general, and having determined that that way is indeed the best we can think of for this specific patient today, we decide to do it, are able to get it done, (practically in a technically good way) and we do so, negotiating as we go with any awkward personnel involved, solving difficult situations and making good judgements about any additional and unexpected problems we find on the spot.

We need to recognize the importance of practical wisdom, but in so doing we need to admit that to exercise this moral reasoning is to exercise a complex capacity which professionals are eternally refining. In so doing they 'carve certainty from uncertainty' (White and Stancombe, 2003, p. 129).

How practical wisdom might be taught and learnt

Practical wisdom can be taught by surgeon educators who respond with sensitivity to the moral issues raised by a given patient's case, and who model this virtue, both in their conduct and in their discussion of the case. It can be developed in the young surgeon by encouragement and a clear indication that it is valued by the teacher. This happens when learners are asked for oral or written evidence: that they recognize what is required at a moral and ethical level in a given and particular patient case; that they are willing to act upon this understanding; and that they do conduct themselves appropriately in respect of this.

Equally, of course, surgical teachers can provide a strong negative model. Those who demonstrate only a technical interest in patients will (inadvertently, perhaps) teach the young surgeon that practical wisdom is not important! This can happen when consultant surgeons themselves engage only in a technical version of deliberation, or do not (appear to) engage in it at all.

A professional judgement

Definition

This is a major decision about action to be taken, which is reached only after careful deliberation which has been enlightened by practical wisdom. It combines the answers to the questions: What ought to be done in this case? What can be done in this case? How shall we go about doing it in this case? It leads into wise action or practice. Aristotle's term for this practice, which is enlightened by practical wisdom, is *praxis*. This is the best action for the circumstances because it is an action which results from reasoning and deliberation.

At the patient consultation stage such a judgement may be reached either with the direct input of the patient, or it may then feed into a more conclusive discussion with the patient, which results in an agreed treatment plan (a final decision about the way forward for this individual patient in the light of his/her context and individuality). Equally, a professional judgement may be a decision about a course of action during the treatment, or it may be the final judgement about how best in a given Trust to go about altering a given policy.

Exploration

An example of this would be a decision which began with a clinical conclusion (reached after the clinical reasoning process), which took account of the context and all the pressures and issues which surrounded it for the individual patient, and which shaped the decision about action, via practical wisdom, to the moral and ethical specifics of the case. Lamond, *et al*,

(1996) would refer to this as a causal judgement, because it is based on the recognition of attributes that explain the problem. At Trust level, in respect of policy matters, for example, the initiating surgeon might have begun with an ideal picture of desired change, but after deliberation and drawing on practical wisdom, would have reached a judgement to argue for setting in motion certain actions that represented the best compromise possible, given the context, circumstances, and personal implications for all employees.

How reaching a professional judgement might be taught and learnt

A professional judgement (decision) and its accompanying wise practice can be taught by taking the entire clinical thinking pathway that has led to it, and making it explicit in discussion or writing.

Indeed, in order to enable teachers and learners to pull the whole of these (sub) processes back into an overall grasp of clinical thinking, we now offer in section two, at Figures 7:3, 7:4, and 7:5, examples of whole thinking pathways, from complex clinical problem setting to final professional judgement.

End notes

1. Surgical teachers should remember that the overall educational aim is to develop young surgeons as independent sources of judgement who can make their own judgements within their own role in the practical setting. They should be self-critical, independent learners, who are also willing to engage in clinical thinking, not only to resolve immediate clinical problems in respect of a given patient, but also to respond to wider professional issues in the service of patients, at the level of public debate and policy making.

2. Learners should bear in mind the following guidance for good decision-making generally.

    ❏ Prioritize tasks, regularly reconsider their order, focus on the decision in hand, always be willing to favour the real emergency.
    ❏ View the problem from a distance, look for inconsistencies, and seek evidence which disproves the decision you are inclined to or habitually favour.
    ❏ Welcome rather than reject uncertainty and recognize the inevitability of complexity (even, suspect that which seems simple).
    ❏ Do not lightly ignore or leave to one side those elements that do not fit your developing decision.
    ❏ Think carefully about the relative significance of elements.
    ❏ Look at the patient (and the clinical thinking pathway) as a whole.
    ❏ Do not rush to identify resemblances between this case and previous ones.

    (See also Kirk and Cox, 2004, p. 146)

3.   In a profession, a tradition of practical reasoning is built up through extending, elaborating and refining the criteria by which actions are to be justified, and showing how these criteria are to be weighed in practical situations. The growth of the tradition is made possible by the collation and discussion of examples of practice, by the insights of gifted individuals and the discovery of new possibilities through experimentation. The result is a formal, accessible body of knowledge, not of a commonsense nature, but of how to engage in effective clinical thinking (see Golby and Parrott, 1999).

4.   Clinical thinking, and all the elements involved in it, can best be developed through processes of reflection. This encourages ways of making meaning out of the thinking process, which recognizes that there may be many points of view and interpretations of the meaning. This is helped by writing as well as talking (see Chapter 5).

5.   We would argue that all these processes can only be developed directly and deliberately in young surgeons from the moment they take on their role and responsibility in the clinical setting as postgraduate doctors. Although we have teased them apart, for the purposes of looking at them more closely, we would in fact wish these processes ultimately to become, in the clinician, part of one holistic approach to good clinical thinking, and enable him/her to take part in the wider policy deliberations as well as the purely clinical.

We would point out that we have construed clinical thinking in the above discussion, as having within it two different forms of professional judgement (judgement as a thinking process and the capacity for thinking), and judgement as a final decision made (judgement as a product). Indeed, there is a third form of knowledge associated with it: namely knowledge of professional judgement at the abstract (metacognitive) level (see Chapter 9).

Education for clinical thinking: three pathways and their educational uses

Below we illustrate three different kinds of complex clinical problems about which surgeons daily have to come to working decisions, and the processes which lead to a wise judgement about action in relation to each of them. We do so in order to assist surgical teachers and learners to begin to see in relation to each of these, the whole pathway of clinical thinking. We believe that there is educational usefulness in these pathways themselves, but that while they remain at the abstract level of a model, they provide only a theoretical purchase on the overall process. We therefore urge readers to explore these ideas and to map onto them their own real-life examples.

The purposes in this are threefold: to explore the use, usefulness and relevance of each pathway in analyzing how surgeons think in different contexts; to encourage readers to critique the pathway in the light of real clinical practice; and to engage surgical teachers and learners in unearthing and critiquing their own particular engagements with clinical thinking.

Figure 7:3 shows the clinical thinking for the most commonly used diagnostic process, of working from patient presentation to agreed treatment plan; Figure 7:4 covers the decisions made during treatment; and Figure 7:5 shows how reasoning and deliberation are used in relation to the wider practical policy issues about which the surgeon needs to decide. In each of these figures we show how the main pathway of clinical thinking presented earlier at Figures 7:1 and 7:2, has to take account of a range of influencing features. The surrounding boxes show the different kinds of influence to be recognized across different pathways.

The first figure, (Figure 7:3), allows us to show how clinical reasoning and deliberation play an equal role in making the professional decision about the initial treatment plan; the second example, (Figure 7:4), shows deliberation as more significant than clinical reasoning, in responding to possible but unexpected clinical features in the treatment pathway; and the third example, (Figure 7:5), illustrates how the wider issues demand deliberation almost to the exclusion of clinical reasoning. This emphasizes to further the irony that traditionally clinical reasoning alone is initiated in medical school and forms the basis for most assessments there, but that in postgraduate clinical practice it is deliberation that plays an increasingly important and central role.

Readers should link each of the three scenarios presented to the generalized features of each relevant pathway model, and then seek their own examples. Readers may at first find it hard to unearth and recognize all the details involved, but it is time well spent because without it there can be no rigour in teaching these processes to learning surgeons, and no means of assessing and recording the learner's achievements in this very important area.

Example one (see Figure 7:3)

The thinking that takes clinicians from a patient's arrival to an agreed treatment plan, together with a generalized comment about the factors to be considered, are presented in the abstract in Figure 7:3. In concrete cases the surgeon needs to take account of the specific processes that affect the construing of the complex clinical problem, the precise factors that feed into the clinical reasoning process, and the particular elements that must be weighed up and adjudicated upon during deliberation on the particular case. The following scenario overleaf offers an example of this.

The scenario of a new outpatient consultation

The context of the case

A female secondary school teacher of forty-eight years is sent to the surgical clinic by her general practitioner (GP), asking for an opinion as to the cause and treatment of her abdominal pain. She has suffered three attacks of pain and on one occasion required admission to hospital whilst on holiday in Spain. Gallstones were identified on ultrasound examination. She is now seeking advice on preventing further attacks of what the GP has diagnosed as biliary colic. She is sent an outpatient appointment in February.

Framing the problem

She is seen in the new outpatient clinic by the Specialist Registrar (SpR) who:

- extracts the salient features from the GP letter;
- begins to think about the possible diagnosis based on his propositional knowledge;
- recalls his previous experience of this condition;
- as a matter of principle holds the presenting diagnosis as questionable;
- has three other key possibilities in mind as to her problem (peptic ulceration, hiatus hernia, or colonic problems).

He thus frames the complex clinical problem as having four diagnostic possibilities which he must place in order of probability.

The clinical reasoning process

He then attempts to make sense of the case by observing the patient, taking a history and critiquing the GP's diagnosis, by recognizing pictures, patterns and signs that will allow him to order his four possibilities.

His observation and the patient's history reveal a fit woman with no co-morbid factors. There has been no history of jaundice. Examination is unremarkable and reveals no abdominal scars.

The diagnosis of biliary colic is the most likely from this evidence. No further tests are deemed necessary and he advises the operation of cholecystectomy by the laparoscopic technique. He takes consent, and prepares the required paperwork necessary to list the patient for the operation. The clinical solution is thus secured.

The scenario of a new outpatient consultation *continued:*

The deliberative process

Before finishing the consultation the patient asks when the operation is likely to take place and how long will she be off work. She says that she is the Head of Department for French and that the final examinations of her students are in June. The registrar tells her that the normal waiting time is about three months and that the Trust requires patients to be treated in the order of listing. She may need to be off work for between three to six weeks depending on recovery. She requests that she has the operation in the school holidays, preferably in August.

The registrar brings in the consultant surgeon to seek his opinion about the patient's request. The consultant talks with the patient and agrees with her to aim to book the operation in August, assuming that no further adverse events occur before that time. In exercising this practical wisdom he has added to the conclusions reached by the SpR and taken account of the feelings and needs of the patient. The consultation is completed and the patient leaves. The consultant talks with the registrar and explains his reasons for making the decisions as he did. The agreed action plan is recorded in the patient's notes.

Comment

This clinical scenario is a common one. It represents the simplest, most easily taught (and by inference easily learned) version of clinical thinking. The processes of clinical decision-making and deliberation are equally balanced in their influence on the case, and they are equally needed, but they have differing roles. It should be noted, too, that the deliberative process here ensures that the patient's needs are fully met, but also that attending to this at the clinical appointment stage should ensure that Trust processes are less likely to unearth confounding factors at a later stage.

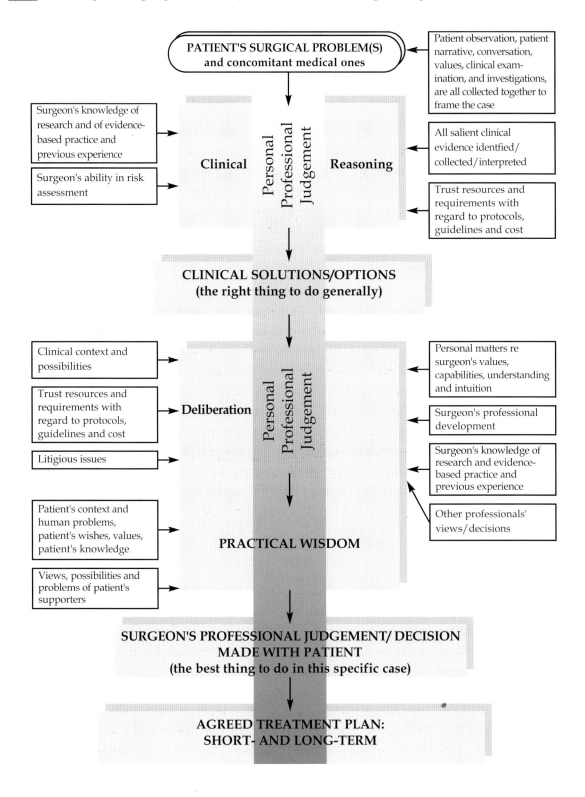

Figure 7:3 The pathway of clinical thinking in a new outpatient consultation.

Example two (see Figure 7:4)

The scenario of new clinical thinking during treatment

The context of the case

A female patient is admitted for laparoscopic cholecystectomy to the day-case unit, which is separate from the main hospital and has no overnight stay beds. She is the first case of the morning and it is anticipated that she will go home in the early evening. The case will be done under general anaesthetic by an experienced specialist registrar assisted by an SHO in surgery. The consultant is available in the theatre suite.

Framing the problem

The patient is anaesthetised, the SpR has inserted the ports and begins the dissection of the gallbladder. The gallbladder is very dilated with omentum stuck to it and there are some patches of necrosis in the wall. The SpR expresses surprise that the case has been listed for day surgery. He begins to mull over the problems of day-case selection for laparoscopic cholecystectomies, and wonders uneasily about the likely logistical problems that will ensue about acquiring a bed for, and transport of, the patient to the main hospital. While thinking this, he proceeds carefully but after half and hour still has not identified the appropriate anatomy to be able to advance the operation. He then realizes that his immediate practical complex clinical problem is to decide whether he can continue with the patient as a day case, and how long he should proceed with the minimally invasive procedure. He is aware of the body language and comment from others in the theatre. The consultant anaesthetist is muttering about case selection, the likely need for an overnight bed and cancelling the rest of the list. The complex clinical problem here is the clinician's, not the patient's!

The clinical reasoning process

The SpR works through in his mind the pros and cons of proceeding with a difficult dissection, which might cause damage to other important structures near the gallbladder. Some of this he shares with the rest of the theatre team. He questions whether it might not be more prudent to convert the operation to an open procedure. He considers the arguments logically, and calculates that there is a case for spending a modest time in further trying to display carefully the anatomy. He also recognizes the disruption that will be caused by failing to do this as a day case not to mention the fact that the department might lose some face in having a second case in two weeks that could not go home on the day of surgery.

The scenario of new clinical thinking during treatment *continued:*

The deliberative process

The SpR calls the consultant surgeon for advice, explaining that he realizes that conversion to an open procedure may be required but he has never before opened a patient listed for day surgery. The consultant scrubs and takes over the case. He confirms the hard stuck nature of the gallbladder and after a total of one hour of surgery makes a decision to convert the procedure to an open cholecystectomy. He directs the scrub nurse to prepare for a change in procedure and requests that things are put in motion to find an in-patient bed as well as to inform the ward medical staff about the change of plan. The theatre staff find the telephone number of the patient's relatives in order that they may be informed of the decision.

The consultant performs a successful open cholecystectomy and the SpR closes the wound. The consultant discusses the case with the SpR and SHO and prepares them for explaining things to the patient. A record of the decisions and actions is made in the patient's notes. As a consequence, one case on the planned list is postponed because of insufficient time to complete the list. Arrangements are put in place for someone to talk to that patient, to explain why this has happened and rebook their operation, putting them first on the list at the next available time. The patient is finally admitted to the ward and discharged five days later after an uncomplicated recovery.

Comment

This scenario demonstrates the need for surgeons to be able to deal with the unexpected. This will require self-knowledge and an ability to think through what is in the best interests of the patient as distinct from those of the surgeon. It will require the surgeon to enact this change and at the same time, maintain the respect and confidence of the theatre team.

There are a number of thoughts and ideas which lie tacitly under the surface of what surgeons actually do. Many of them are easily attended to by senior surgeons almost on auto-pilot, without the need to focus in detail on them. But inexperienced surgeons, who have not learnt to explore their clinical thinking rigorously and so not developed an orderly mind in respect of their thought processes, may become lost in the mists of competing demands, and fail to recognize, focus on and act upon the most significant of them. Here, the most significant was recognizing and doing the right thing for the patient in a timely manner.

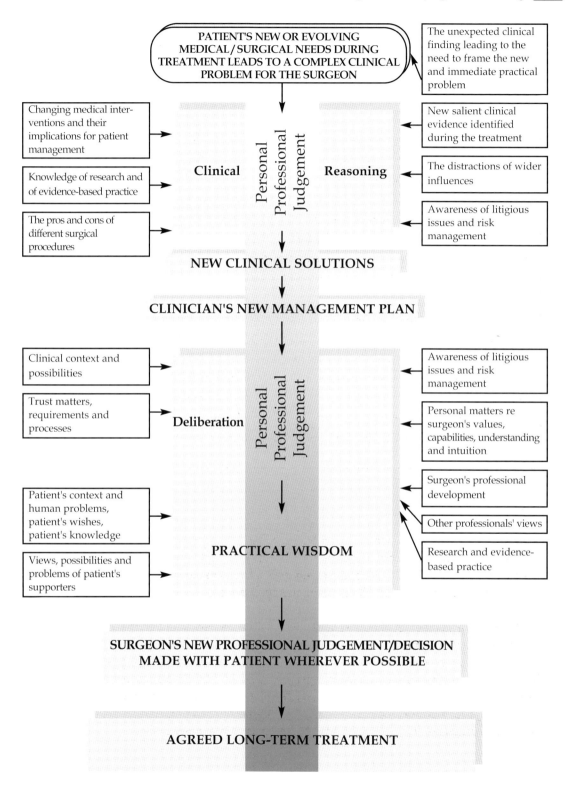

Figure 7:4 The pathway of clinical thinking during treatment.

Example three (see Figure 7:5)

A scenario of the wider issues of clinical practice

The context of the case

It is the 14th of August and the ward medical staff are new. A patient is on the operating list for abdominal aortic aneurysm surgery the following morning and is waiting at home for the call to be told that there is a suitable bed available. He has already been cancelled by the Trust once because of bed problems. The critical care unit now has a patient with methicillin-resistant *Staphylococcus aureus* (MRSA) in her wound and five other patients have become contacts. The unit is full with respect to the number of critical care staff available to nurse the patients.

Framing the problem

MRSA is a recurring problem in the Trust. There is a new Trust policy in place that the bed manager discusses the case with the Trust lead for MRSA who is a consultant microbiologist. This is done and the bed manager offers a solution that arrangements could be made to 'special' the patient on the surgical ward, which is clean. This is accepted. The ward medical staff are informed and the patient is phoned and advised to come into the hospital. There is a sense of relief that another cancellation of this particular patient will be avoided. The consultant vascular surgeon finds out about this arrangement at eight o'clock on the day of surgery, when he does a pre-operative visit. His problem now is: does he accept these arrangements or overrule them?

The clinical reasoning process

The patient's needs for an operation have not changed but the resources available have. The need for a critical care bed is essential. It is the surgeon's responsibility to ensure a suitable post-operative bed is available for his patient before the operation is started. The risks of infection with MRSA to this patient include the risk of death. As the clinical solution to this, the surgeon cancels the case, but the underlying problems remain. The patient still needs to be found a suitable bed and the risky Trust policy will, without some intervention, continue. What should the consultant now do?

A scenario of the wider issues of clinical practice *continued:*

The deliberative process

He recognizes that he has fulfilled his responsibilities to the patient in this particular context but there is an urgent need to explore and change the Trust MRSA policy. His heart sinks, as he knows that this will incur more meetings, diplomacy and time. He gathers his thoughts into an argument that will persuade non-surgeons to change the protocol. This involves his knowledge of his professional responsibilities, Trust systems and policies, Trust personnel, and the current spotlight in which MRSA is being discussed in the media. He talks to the key members of staff involved and a meeting is set up to review the protocols. The particular aim is to ensure that the protocol indicates that the consultant in charge of the case is informed of such problems before the patient is admitted.

Comment

There is no direct patient participation needed in this case either with respect to his condition or his wishes. The clinical decision made previously is not in dispute. The process of deliberation is the main thrust of this scenario.

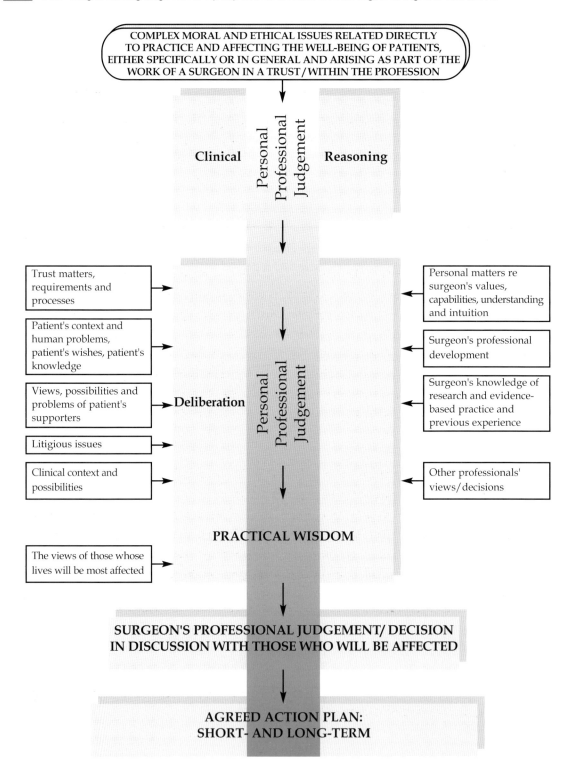

Figure 7:5 The pathway of clinical thinking for attending to the wider issues of clinical practice.

The importance of revisiting decisions and thinking at all stages

We have presented the pathways in linear fashion, but would strongly emphasize the fact that in real practice, clinicians will always revisit the decisions and the thinking that led to them, when elements that do not fit emerge. This will be especially so when the diagnosis at the end of the clinical reasoning pathway is still somewhat uncertain. The first decision being made at this point enables the progression of care of the patient, but is not necessarily the final diagnosis.

The following example illustrates this.

Case scenario

A 28-year-old male presents to the acute hospital A & E department on Christmas Day. His symptoms are of acute pain in both calves, he is unable to walk and feels extremely unwell. Clinical examination reveals hypotension, thin thready pulses, upper limb peripheral cyanosis, tense calves, impalpable pulses in the feet but with capilliary return in the toes. On receiving the blood results which demonstrate acidosis and renal failure, and urine demonstrating rhabdomyosis, a diagnosis of acute renal failure and bilateral calf compression syndrome is made. The precise initiating cause of this at this point is unclear. Steps are put in place to begin treatment of the renal failure initiating renal dialysis, and arrangements made to decompress the muscle compartments in both calves.

Twelve hours later his condition has deteriorated further, and further clinical reasoning takes place to re-frame the problem and to continue to find an initial cause. There is developing a strong intuitive sense (based on experience) that his heart may be the primary dysfunctional organ. There is strong need for the clinicians to hold open the final framing of the clinical problem, and to continue to revise their clinical reasoning, alongside further investigations. These include, in addition to blood tests and clinical monitoring, ultrasound imaging of the heart and peripheral vessels.

Comment

Where at any stage uncertainty remains about the accuracy of diagnosis, recycling through the pathway must always be carried out.

End note

Equipped with a grasp of the whole field of clinical thinking, and an understanding of the elements and processes within it, and enlightened by the above clinical examples, we can now turn in the following chapter to the assessment of the learning surgeon's clinical thinking. Initially (for a learner in an early attachment) this may be carried out in respect of the individual sections of the process, and then put together as a whole. More experienced learners may well, from the start, be able to focus on the whole of each pathway (as shown earlier). Learning surgeons with problems in one area may nonetheless need to return to one aspect. For these reasons we shall treat them separately in the following chapter.

Chapter 8

Assessing clinical thinking

Introduction

This chapter provides the detail of ways of assessing the clinical thinking of learning surgeons, which in Chapter 7 above, we present as the central core of surgical practice. In doing so it adds detail and richness to the concepts introduced in that chapter.

Relationship to previous chapter

Whilst we would not normally support the disengagement of assessment from teaching and learning (believing them to be parts of one whole, and seeing assessment as fundamentally supportive to education, as discussed in Chapter 6), we have on this occasion split the assessment of clinical thinking from its development as offered in Chapter 7, simply to prevent the latter from being of an unwieldy size. Readers are therefore urged to treat this as the final section of the previous chapter, and to read that first. They are also referred back to Chapter 6 for an overview of assessment and its educational purposes, and for the definitions of technical terms like summative and formative assessment.

The uses of these assessment processes

Given the significance of clinical thinking, it is surprising that until now, evidence of ability in it has not been a central requirement of assessment for the learning surgeon. We note with interest that by comparison to this, members of other professions, who wish to be formally recognized as advanced practitioners, have to engage in learning about and developing their clinical thinking, through postgraduate courses. We believe that the same requirement to develop clinical thinking should be true for postgraduates in medicine and surgery.

We cannot stress too strongly, however, that the processes we offer in this chapter are not suitable (indeed, we would argue that no assessment process is suitable) for use as a one-off test, to identify and eject from the system a failing trainee.

Rather, assessment, including self-assessment, which is always the ultimate goal of good education, can be used in a variety of ways, almost all of them developmental, to promote the learning of clinical thinking. At the start of learners' careers (or the start of an attachment), learners can engage in self-assessment (in the form of a learning-needs analysis), and surgical teachers can engage in informal assessment (in the shape of an induction conversation with the learner about this). This can be used to chart learners' baseline understanding of, capacity for, and ability in, clinical thinking. At relevant points throughout the learner's career, assessment can provide ways of analyzing and developing the clinical thinking that lies beneath the learner's maturing clinical actions. (These points can be chosen during an attachment, either as the teacher's professional judgement directs, or as the learner chooses, in order to place evidence of achievement on record.) Here, assessment can focus on the overall process (following a whole pathway of the kind offered at 7:3, 7:4, and 7:5), or attend to a specific aspect in which the learner has shown a weakness. At the end of an attachment, or programme, a summative assessment of clinical thinking can be placed on record.

The ultimate intention of all this is to develop the learner to the point where their clinical thinking is fluent, dependable and of mature professional standard, when the main headings of the overall pathway are used merely as an *aide mémoire*, and when there is further recourse to the assessment details only to help unravel a special and complex case. If, despite help offered, and numerous opportunities and warnings, the learner still makes no progress in developing these elements into a whole fluent clinical thinking process, then, and then alone, will the use of these assessment processes already have generated enough evidence to identify and act upon failure.

Recognizing, surfacing and tracing clinical thinking

The abilities to be developed

Clinical thinking is of course both invisible and tacit. This makes it difficult to recognize, make visible, trace, explore, learn and assess. The intentions of this chapter are to offer teachers and learners ways of surfacing, making explicit and critiquing their thinking, and to show how it can be assessed both formatively (so that it can be developed further) and summatively (so that the learner's achievement can be recorded). Indeed, we would urge that some formal records are kept of the learner's development of clinical thinking in each attachment, which can then be used as the basis of a final, summative assessment.

In order to provide such evidence, it is crucial that learners first develop the ability to trace and make overt the tacit thinking that underlies their clinical actions and decisions, and then offer a critique of it (by reference back to the pathways offered in Chapter 7). Recognizing, surfacing and tracing clinical thinking will initially demand thoughtful practice by learners and their teachers. Because of its importance, we offer an example later in this chapter.

Once learning surgeons can do this, they will be able to demonstrate the following facility and knowledge at appropriate points during their learning:

- ☐ facility and fluency in the overall processes of clinical thinking;
- ☐ a knowledge of, and the ability to use intelligently, the processes of problem setting, clinical reasoning, and deliberation (including practical wisdom).

They will need to do this both by giving an account of them within their everyday practice, and by demonstrating the visible signs of them in their conduct with patients and colleagues. The capacity for personal professional judgement and the quality of the final professional decision will also need to be identified in these formative and summative assessments, in the learners' general conduct during service commitments, and particularly in the assessment of technical and surgical procedures as shown in Chapter 10.

The role of narrative in providing a basis for assessment

We have indicated that reflective narratives (either oral or written) are an important means of attending to the invisible elements beneath surgical practice. We argued this in Chapter 7 (particularly in respect of clinical thinking), and in Chapter 5 (more generally in respect of the important role of reflection in learning and assessment).

Clinical thinking is probably the most deeply tacit of all elements that make up the thinking surgeon. The best way of unearthing it is to launch into the construction of a reflective narrative (attending, of course, to the normal requirements to render the event anonymous). This will aid both the recognition and overt surfacing of the thinking processes. Every attempt of learners to do this will generate material that can be assessed. Usefully, that which is generated informally in a teaching situation, as a means of informing teacher and learner of the learner's growth of understanding of clinical thinking, can itself - if chosen to be placed on formal record - become a formal element of summative assessment. Such a formal assessment will chart a learner's developing grasp of the thinking processes, together with his/her increasing ability to capture and explore them.

Constructing a narrative to demonstrate understanding and critique of clinical thinking

Ironically, the most important activity in constructing a narrative as the basis for assessment of clinical thinking, is simply to get started on a story which leads up to a clinical conclusion or a professional judgement.

Once started, the processes of thinking, talking and writing about the actions will gain an impetus of their own and lead the practitioner to uncover more of what lay under the events than s/he was aware of at the time. The processes are as follows.

❑ Seek to construct the story just as it is remembered (doing so as soon as possible after it has happened).

❑ Start with the facts (these are fairly easily told orally).

❑ Write them down in the correct order as far as memory allows.

❑ If it is helpful, map them onto the appropriate pathway found in Chapter 7.

❑ Get help and prompting about the facts from others who were present.

❑ Add in brackets, behind each fact captured, the detail of the thinking which underlay your actions (do this in another colour or font and number the points).

❑ Look at the thinking processes you have surfaced so far, and enrich the facts you have captured, so as to make your actions more explicit.

❑ Go backwards and forwards between the facts about your actions and the thinking that you recognize beneath their surface, using each to critique and expand the other.

❑ Work over these and keep refining and adding the details as you remember them.

❑ Keep working over the chronological order.

❑ Use the pathways offered in the previous chapter to help you distinguish between various kinds of thinking and to offer a critique of the clinical thinking engaged in.

❑ Write the critique at the end of your narrative, using the numbered points to identify the elements you are discussing.

An example

The following example comes from a very early piece of writing of this kind by a consultant, who merely offers the story of her actions and does not unearth her underlying thinking.

Case scenario: version one

Cancelling a patient's operation on the day of surgery

It takes more than just knowing about the condition and being able to do the operation.

The case

It was a Tuesday morning at 8am and I arrived to review the patients on my all-day operating list. The previous Friday I had reviewed the list and it showed a patient with an abdominal aortic aneurysm from my vascular waiting list and two patients from the common waiting list for thyroid surgery. On the Monday I had been working away from the Trust. Late on the previous Friday, one of the patients listed for thyroid surgery had phoned to cancel their operation because of a concurrent medical problem. In order not to miss the operating space a patient requiring recurrent incisional hernia surgery was given the place left by the cancellation. This new patient was admitted to the ward on the Monday and consented by the trainees ready for theatre on the Tuesday. I enquired why another thyroid patient had not been added and was told that this patient was next on the list. I visited the patient for the hernia repair on the ward. His case notes were very thick and were being read very carefully by the consultant anaesthetist. I observed that the patient walked with a stick and he told me that he was very disabled with joint problems. After a short conversation with him it seemed to me that both he and I were less informed than we should be about his surgical problem. This was my first knowledge of him. His understanding of the possible post-operative events that might complicate his recovery was very limited. I made the decision to postpone his case and arranged to see him again the following Friday in my outpatient clinic. There was a feeling abroad that I was over-reacting.

Note that this outline story is quite short, and took no more than ten minutes to write. Note too, that nowhere in this story is the complex clinical problem stated in clear and simple terms, but it certainly lies implicit beneath the surface. In other words it is still tacit at this stage. How and at what point should it be made explicit? Before reading further, readers might wish to try to trace the clinical thinking involved here, and even to identify the points in the story where the facts themselves will need elaboration.

This story is typical of what experts will offer about their practice when asked to explain it. Indeed, quite possibly in the working lives of most senior clinicians, their formulation of the initiating complex clinical problem is never (and never needs to be) stated overtly. Yet precision of formulation is crucial to shaping the rest of the decisions and actions about treatment. In the past, facility in this used to grow in the learning surgeon during long and close working relationships with the consultant. Now, the shorter time available for the education of surgeons does not allow for this. The learning surgeon thus needs to be helped more quickly to recognize the need for, to understand the processes of, and to gain expertise and rigour in, such precise formulation. Surgical teachers need therefore to be articulate about these matters in their explanation (of some) of their practice.

The story above is an example of the difficulty of exhuming this deeply buried tacit knowledge, and of the attention that needs to be given to it by teaching surgeons in painstakingly surfacing and exploring their practice in preparation for supporting the learner.

Below, is the same story, which has now been worked on for half an hour by the consultant with a view to unearthing the thinking and decision-making within it. The comments in bold type identify the kind of thinking which underlay the actions reported. The numbers against these allow for expansion of these points in a critique beneath the narrative. The italics show some examples of how the original narrative was extended by considering the clinical thinking that ran beneath the action and recognizing the need to elaborate on the thinking in the story. It will also be noted that she has reshaped the written presentation to emphasize the various stages of the action and thought.

Case scenario: version two

Cancelling a patient's operation on the day of surgery

It takes more than just knowing about the condition and being able to do the operation.

The case

It was a Tuesday morning at 8am and I arrived to review the patients on my all-day operating list. The previous Friday I had reviewed the list and it showed a patient with an abdominal aortic aneurysm from my vascular waiting list and two patients from the common waiting list for thyroid surgery. On the Monday I had been working away from the Trust. Late on the previous Friday, one of the patients listed for thyroid surgery had phoned to cancel their operation because of a concurrent medical problem. In order not to miss the operating space a patient requiring recurrent incisional hernia surgery was given the place left by the cancellation. **(1 complex clinical problem beginning to emerge.)** This new patient had been admitted to the ward on the Monday **(2 complex clinical problem shaping up as conflicting needs of patient, Trust, and learners.)** He had been consented by the trainees ready for theatre on the Tuesday. *I recognized that overruling a decision made by learners might not be good for them, but the patient's interests had to come first. I made a mental note to talk them through this later.* **(3 complex clinical problem is formulated as: to operate or not on the hernia patient).** *I did not make this explicit in my initial version of the narrative.*

I enquired why another thyroid patient had not been added *because the type of surgery and fitness of the patient would have made for a more straightforward operation with a thyroid patient than a patient admitted with an incisional hernia. This mattered because of the length of time available on the list, the need to appraise the hernia patient of the risks, and my not having seen the hernia patient before. I was told that this patient was next on the list.* **(4a clinical reasoning takes account of Trust demands).** I visited the patient for

---

Cancelling a patient's operation on the day of surgery (version two) *continued:*

the hernia repair on the ward **(4b clinical reasoning takes account of all that can be gained from meeting the patient.)** His case notes were very thick **(4c clinical reasoning takes account of extent of co-morbid problems)** and were being read very carefully by the consultant anaesthetist. **(4d clinical reasoning takes account of the concerns of other colleagues.)** I observed that the patient walked with a stick **(4e clinical reasoning takes account of observation of patient. 5 Now the clinical solution is becoming clear - not to operate at this time -** *I did not note this initially in my narrative)* and he told me that he was very disabled with joint problems. **(6a deliberation includes as a factor the priority of patient's other problems and personal story.)** After a short conversation with him it seemed to me that both he and I were less informed **(6b, and c deliberation takes account of how the patient might be seeing his problem, and the patient's resulting needs)** than we should be about his surgical problem. This was my first knowledge of him. **(6d deliberation takes account of the practitioner's knowledge.)** His understanding of the possible post-operative events that might complicate his recovery was very limited. **(6e deliberation takes account of the need to educate the patient to understand the risks and to have time to assimilate them. 7 practical wisdom highlights the recognition of my moral responsibilities to the patient, and the need to act accordingly).**

I made the decision to postpone his case **(8 professional judgement)** and arranged to see him again the following Friday in my outpatient clinic **(8 professional judgement and agreed action plan).** There was a feeling abroad that I was over-reacting **(9 I now recognize overtly that there is a need to be able to explain my thinking in detail to a number of affected parties).**

Critique

Clearly, points 1 and 2 lead up to the emergence of the complex clinical problem at point 3. As a learner I would expect to work on giving voice (in my head) to a more precise formulation of such problems. This problem is complex because endemic to it are competing arguments and priorities leading to different solutions.

Points 4a to 4e show the clinical elements considered, and the reasoning used about them. I could have said more about the logic with which I ordered these points, and as a learner would try to do so in future. Point 5 shows the clinical solution arising from these arguments. If I needed to review this solution it would be important to be able to set out and explore the logic of my clinical reasoning.

Points 6a to 6e show how this clinical solution is deliberated about. It shows that I recognize a number of different points of view (none of them easily prioritized), but it does not show how I go about doing this. Point 7 shows that I recognize my moral responsibilities to the patient, and respond to the patient's needs. Point 8 offers the professional judgement and agreed treatment plan. In point 9 I have recognized overtly some other moral obligations which spring from this event.

Once the learning surgeon can do this comfortably, s/he is ready to provide evidence, when needed, of the first of the two areas listed above (facility and fluency in the overall process of clinical thinking). The second area was knowledge of and ability to use intelligently the processes of clinical problem framing, clinical reasoning and professional judgement (including practical wisdom). Ways of assessing these - or the parts of them as needed - are now set out below.

Assessing the processes of framing the complex clinical problem

Assessment of the factors that influence how the problem is framed

We referred above to those attributes of the learning surgeon that affect how s/he construes the complex clinical problem. These are the personal theories, beliefs, assumptions, and values, together with professional values, which make up that surgeon's prevailing view of the world. We noted that they cause him/her to see life through lenses shaped by his/her autobiography and personality. Self-awareness is an important factor here. It is to be hoped too, that the surgeon will be able to make the leap into the patient's shoes and see the case through his/her lenses. Here, imagination would be being displayed. Further, the willingness of the learner to recognize how other colleagues might construe the problem and why, would demonstrate a consciousness of the multi-professional dimension in all clinical work.

The learning surgeon's awareness of these issues, together with a recognition that problems are not 'given' but are construed by professionals (with the possibility that they might be construed differently by different practitioners) should surface in any narrative (oral or written) of a successful surgeon who is asked to show achievement in this kind of problem setting.

In addition to this, of course, such a surgeon would need to provide evidence at both formative and summative stages that s/he was aware of and able to utilize the following processes. Evidence of them can be supplied by the learner either orally or in writing, but this would need to be confirmed also by observations of the visible elements of the learning surgeon's conduct by colleagues, patients and official teachers.

Assessment of the processes for framing the initial complex clinical problem

All pathways, as illustrated in Figures 7:3, 7:4, and 7:5, start with the need for the surgeon to frame the complex clinical problem. The details involved in this framing-up process will be different for each pathway. Table 8:1 offers the details for each pathway that can be used by surgeons to engage in the framing process. The table is not designed so that the columns can be read across. They merely list in order for each pathway the explorative activities which the learning surgeon needs to engage in. The relevant part of the table could be used as a checklist for framing a problem within a given pathway (though not as a tick box list, as in the assessment of competencies, since what are offered here are not skills).

Table 8:1 Points for exploration in framing the complex clinical problem for the purposes of assessment.

Within diagnostic reasoning (Fig 7:3)	Within the treatment pathway (Fig 7:4)	Within the policy pathway (Fig 7:5)
Patient's presenting diagnosis	Whose problem it is? (patient's or clinician's?)	Growing awareness of an incomplete or inappropriate resource for patient care
The range of possible diagnoses for this disease	The unexpected event which signals this problem	The event which pointed out this problem
The clinician's previous experience of this problem (though this case may be different)	That which has led to this state of affairs (predictable or unpredictable)?	That which has led to this state of affairs
How questionable is the presenting diagnosis?	The reasons that might be possible for the event	The possible reasons for it
The patient's demeanour and physical features (observation)	Previous experience of this problem (but this case may be different)	Previous experience of this problem (but remember this example may be different)
The patient's overall story	Whether these are urgent or secondary to the immediate need to identify the present, practical problem	State the present, urgent, practical problem as you now frame it
The significant signs	State the problem as you now frame it	How can the immediate problem be clarified?
Differential diagnosis	What will conduce to the solution of the immediate practical problem?	What will conduce to the solution?
The critique that could be made of the presenting diagnosis		
State the problem as you now frame it		
What will conduce to clarifying and confirming the resultant diagnosis?		

These processes can be assessed by oral discussion between teacher and learner, which focuses on real examples provided either by the teacher or the learner.

Assessing the processes of clinical reasoning

Assessment of the foundation strategies for clinical reasoning

The learning surgeon can build a foundation of strategies and tactics for use in clinical reasoning, and these can also profitably be assessed in cases where learners are showing weakness in this area, by setting up written and oral activities that focus on the detail of these. Cohn (1989) offers advice of this kind to other health care professionals. We have adapted her lists of activities and strategies, which are crucial to successful practice (Table 8:2).

Table 8:2 Activities and strategies, which are crucial to successful practice.

The successful learning surgeon:

- notes examples of when routine treatment fits easily and when it does not;
- develops awareness of the different kinds of diagnostic categories;
- builds a mental library of patient stories;
- clusters observations and develops pattern recognition;
- develops hypotheses as a routine even in situations when they are not the responsible clinician;
- builds a foundation for testing the assumptions on which these hypotheses are based;
- confronts the key obstacles in making these 'stick';
- seeks for and responds to the unexpected at all points in the clinical reasoning;
- explores the impact of particular treatment on patients;
- reformulates initial plans;
- reasons in new ways (uses narrative approaches, and interpersonal perspectives);
- 'chunks' information;
- asks probing questions at key choice points.

Cohn offers too, in a list at the end of her paper, the following strategies for learning clinical reasoning. The following represents her advice to learners to gain:

- ❐   repeated experience with patients with a similar diagnosis;
- ❐   repeated interaction with the same patient over several weeks;
- ❐   observation of patient/doctor interactions (observe with a purpose);

- a repertoire of stories, by sharing with peers and teachers;
- insight into an interesting individual case by writing a detailed study of the patient (anonymizing it, of course).

Following Cox, we would also advise learners to develop the following rule-of-thumb knowledge.

- Know what to look for (what kind of knowledge to draw upon).
- Search for evidence of cause.
- Interpret what is found and infer explanations.
- Intuitively recognize patterns of disease or of aberrant details.
- Choose investigations that will differentiate between diagnoses.
- Discriminate between similar clinical pictures produced by different diseases.
- Judge when enough evidence is at hand.
- Scan all body systems systematically for symptoms or signs of malfunction.

(See Cox, 1999, pp. 84-94.)

He also makes the point that there are six ways that doctors understand patients' problems. We advise learners to use this list as an *aide mémoire* in their work and to show evidence of it during both formative and summative assessment. The six ways are:

- doctors' sensory and perceptual repertoire (seeing, hearing, feeling and smelling);
- their verbal and semantic repertoire (patient's talk, doctor's clarification);
- their logical repertoire (reasoning how pieces fit together);
- their numerical repertoire (calculation, probability, and prediction);
- their affective repertoire (interpersonal reactions and emotions);
- their prescriptive repertoire (what can be done in a case like this).

(adapted from Cox, 1999, p. 137.)

All these lists indicate areas of possible discussion and explanation between teacher and learner on assessment occasions that are informal or formal, formative or summative.

Assessment of the key processes of clinical reasoning

We would argue, following the work of Higgs (1990), and our own explorations, that there are five main processes within clinical reasoning, all of which call to a greater or lesser extent on personal judgement. They are: the collection of evidence; identifying the salient factors in this evidence; distilling the meaning from the clinical evidence; coming to a clinical decision (conclusion); and planning treatment in the light of the clinical conclusion. Table 8:3 offers the detail of these key processes, for use in informal and formal assessment exercises.

Table 8:3 Key processes in clinical reasoning.

Processes	Overall activity	Detail
Process 1	Collect the evidence	Observe patient Converse and establish rapport with patient Take patient's history Listen to patient narrative, focusing on key issues Examine patient Appropriately investigate patient Communicate with other relevant people
Process 2	Identify the salient factors in process one	
Process 3	Distil the meaning of the clinical evidence	Draw on: the salient factors identified in process 2 all relevant propositional knowledge research findings where relevant experiential knowledge contextual information about the patient and their inter-dependents familiarity with the Trust as an organization and its requirements and resources
Process 4	Coming to a clinical decision/conclusion	Identify main problem Determine a working hypothesis Make a working diagnosis Make a plan for care Defend decision
Process 5	Designing a treatment plan in the light of the clinical decision	Re-assess treatment criteria Choose between alternative treatments Provide relief or deal with cause Consider short- and long-term management

Learners need to be aware of and competent in these processes. They need to be aware of, to think about, and be able to report on (show evidence of) their judgements in relation to:

☐ the validity and reliability of information received;
☐ the sequence, type, amount, duration, of questions related to:
  • the expected findings;
  • test specificity and sensitivity;
  • effects on the patient of evidence collection;
  • the significance of the findings in relation to the hypothesis.
☐ the fluency and saliency of their thinking and how well it leads to efficient action;
☐ a critical review of own knowledge base and skills (including interpersonal reasoning) and input into, or reorganization of, own knowledge base.

The quality of the learning surgeon's clinical reasoning will need to be assessed using the professional judgement of the assessing surgeon or other competent professional. In addition to this, we believe, with Higgs, that learners can (to an extent) self-assess in many of these processes. This would, however, need to be corroborated by colleagues in the inter-professional team (focusing on the processes listed above) because learners can have a mistaken impression of their abilities (their own judgement might be faulty). Processes in which learners should be encouraged to develop self-assessment are:

☐ collection of data;
☐ interpersonal skills in data collection;
☐ interpersonal skills in decision-making;
☐ knowledge base (scope/content);
☐ knowledge base (organization);
☐ knowledge base (accessibility);
☐ cognitive skills (reasoning/logic);
☐ cognitive skills (intuition/lateral thinking/creative thinking);
☐ cognitive skills (hypothesis testing and generation);
☐ skills in critical evaluation and review of these processes (skills in metacognition and in critical self-evaluation).

Chapter 9 attends in more detail to issues related to the knowledge base.

Assessing the processes of deliberation

The processes of deliberation can, to an extent, be made overt between the teacher and learner in the clinical setting, and by this means the learner can be helped to extend what is considered salient. However, it should be recognized that in deliberation there are some elements that are logical (considering the branching pathways of pros and cons) and some that are an inevitable complex amalgam of weighing many issues, not every part of which can be recognized and made known.

For this reason, the quality of the learning surgeon's deliberations can be assessed by making as overt as possible the processes by which s/he unearthed what to consider, considered it and came to a judgement. Quality here might involve the learner showing awareness of the complexity and inevitably tangled nature of some elements.

We believe with Grundy 1987, p. 65, that: 'Deliberation incorporates processes of interpretation and making meaning of a situation so that appropriate action can be decided upon and taken.' We would argue that deliberative thinking draws on personal judgement in the following processes:

- critiquing the clinical decision (working diagnosis);
- seeking out and considering carefully any unexpected or easily ignored elements which do not fit the working diagnosis;
- recognizing and allowing for the ambiguities of the individual case;
- recognizing the full range of pressures on the particular patient case;
- recognizing the patient's entire context and perspectives;
- listening to the practitioner's intuition;
- attending to wider pattern recognition and scanning the whole;
- taking account of the views and knowledge of colleagues;
- taking account of the resources (constraints and possibilities) of the Trust;
- taking account of the Trust and Government managerial demands (including targets);
- scrutinizing honestly the clinician's own values, humanity, and abilities.

Deliberation often requires revisiting a situation and therefore putting in more effort to solving the problem. It looks beyond the evidence provided by clinical reasoning. It also involves:

- a properly disinterested interest in the patient;
- the willingness by the clinician to 'go the second mile';
- taking a step back (and viewing patterns from a distance);
- not letting self-interest of the clinician or Trust affect the decision.

Ultimately such deliberation can also be assessed in the assessment of professional judgement, which the learner formulates at the end of the process (see below).

Assessing the learning surgeon's processes of professional judgement

As Golby and Parrott point out: 'Many different sorts of understanding must come together in any overall judgement in the service of a client' and professionals' practical judgements on the individual cases set before them will always be made in the light of 'an ideal of service'. That is to say, they will have in mind a notion of what constitutes a reasonable and achievable good for that client so far as their service is concerned' (Golby and Parrott, 1999, p. 25).

Our understanding of professional judgement is based on Aristotelian thinking. Here, the practitioner engages in a kind of active practical enquiry, which has a moral thrust in that it is concerned with determining what should be done for the best in a practical situation. This is in opposition to theoretical (scientific) enquiry, which seeks to establish truths about the world or to speculate neutrally on how things are ordered (see Carr 1995, pp. 68-73). We believe that the important components of professional judgement are the thought processes involved in the judgement (the questions posed; the factors taken account of during, and central to, deliberation; the role of theory; and the justification for action).

Having understood the practical situation as far as possible by exploring it thoroughly through asking questions and identifying factors and engaging in reasoning about them, the practitioner, guided by personal judgement, chooses an action (which is the visible enactment of the judgement). During this process, theory provides a guide, not a specific direction. In determining the quality of the learner's professional judgement in order to facilitate the development of it, it is necessary to examine the role that theory has played. In characterizing the quality of the professional judgement, all these matters need to be attended to.

Introducing Table 8:4 for the assessment of professional judgement

Table 8:4 offers a means of categorizing the quality of the professional judgement made by the learning surgeon. In assessing the learner's professional judgement, this table can be used in conjunction with the following questions, which learners can pose for themselves, or in which surgical teachers can assess learning surgeons whose judgements they are uneasy about.

Summary of questions to use with the table

The questions in Table 8:5 can be used to prompt the learner to explore thoroughly their thinking processes, beginning at the point where the clinical conclusion has been reached and leading up to and including the final professional judgement. Surgical teachers may wish to use these orally with learners, or to encourage learners to use them to practise self-assessment of their own judgement-making.

Table 8:4 Understanding the kinds of judgement that surgeons might make. With acknowledgement to the work of Fish and Coles, 1998, pp. 280-281.

THOUGHT PROCESSES INVOLVED IN JUDGEMENT

Kind of judgement surgeons might make	Question posed	Factors and processes central to deliberation	Role of theory	Justification for action	Visible response (action resulting from judgement)	Characterization of judgement
Hasty judgements Not thought through	None	Ideas randomly chosen (no saliency) and/or inappropriately processed	None	None	Knee-jerk reaction	Unsatisfactory response Unprofessional
Habitual judgements Very poorly thought through	None ("I've seen this before. This is what is done")	No factors selected, no deliberation involved. Aim only for quick decision	Not recognized as important	Not clearly thought out (but might be able to be justified *post hoc*)	Reacts in habitual way	Automatic reflex/response Practitioner as automaton
Tactical judgements Based on copying	What would my seniors do?	Factors/reasoning based on seniors' practice and actions - without critique	Theory confirms actions, but theory not considered critically	*Post hoc* using others' arguments	Selects tactics known to be approved by senior staff	Practical response Practitioner as apprentice

Continued:

Table 8:4 *continued* **Understanding the kinds of judgement that surgeons might make. With acknowledgement to the work of Fish and Coles 1998, pp. 280-281.**

THOUGHT PROCESSES INVOLVED IN JUDGEMENT

Kind of judgement surgeons might make	Question posed	Factors and processes central to deliberation	Role of theory	Justification for action	Visible response (action resulting from judgement)	Characterization of judgement
Strategic judgements Based on own interest	What am *I* able to do now and how will *I* do that?	Salient factors recognized. Practitioner's reasoning related to what s/he can do, and endpoint set to fit what s/he can do	Theory enlightens practice and is enlightened by it but only in respect of means (not ends)	Justification based on personal ideas and actions	Considers own personal abilities and picks way forward assuming endpoint is fixed	Considered response Practitioner as senior technician
Professional insightful judgements Based on holistic view of event	What is in the patient's best interests? What can I offer? What else is relevant?	All salient factors selected. Full deliberative processes used. Moral and ethical questions raised about competing moral ideals and dilemmas	Practitioner makes meanings out of (theorizes) practice and the relationship between theory and practice	Justification through both deliberative and reflective processes	Active practical enquiry about what should be done for the best in this case, able to do it, and does it	Enlightened response Practitioner as enlightened professional, working on the basis of practical wisdom

Table 8:5 Questions to prompt the learner.

In coming to your professional judgement at the end of the clinical thinking process:

What questions did you ask yourself?

Possible answers/observations:
> None
> What would my seniors do?
> What can I do now and get on with?
> What is in the patient's best interest and what can I offer?

What factors did you take account of?

Possible answers/observations:
> Ideas chosen randomly
> None
> Factors seniors would pin-point
> Salient factors related to my abilities
> All salient factors

What processes of thought did you use?

Possible answers/observations:
> Inappropriate processes
> Drive for quick decision
> Reasoning my seniors would use
> Reasoning related to what I can do
> Full deliberative process

What theoretical basis has your decision? (role of theory in decision-making)

Possible answers/observations:
> None
> Theory not important
> Theory confirms actions afterwards
> Theory thought about before and after (but only in respect of how to do things)
> Formal theory, personal theory and theory made out of practice called upon at all points and in respect of both how to do something and whether it should be done at all

How would you justify your subsequent action?

Possible answers/observations:
> Not sure
> Muddled thinking
> By use of others' arguments
> Justification based on personal ideas
> Justification through offering deliberative and reflective processes.

Answers should be related to Table 8.4

Having established the importance of surgeons' thinking, we can now turn to the knowledge base that this thinking draws upon.

Exploring the knowledge base of surgical practice

Introduction

New perspectives on knowledge, and the nature of practice knowledge
Not knowing what one does not know
Re-orienting our view of knowledge
Other ways of construing the divisions of knowledge
Ways of knowing in the arts and sciences
Ways of knowing in professional practice
The components of practice knowledge
Mapping practice knowledge for professionals generally

The practice knowledge of surgeons and how to teach and assess it
The sources of practice knowledge for surgeons
Mapping the components of knowledge that surgeons use in practice
How surgeons use knowledge differently at different learning stages
Focusing on the knowledge used in clinical thinking
The scenario of a new outpatient consultation
The scenario of new clinical thinking during treatment
The scenario of the wider issues of clinical practice

End note

Introduction

It is our unashamed intention in this chapter, to challenge and re-shape surgeons' understanding of the nature of knowledge generally, and of the role of knowledge in their professional practice specifically. We therefore seek to demonstrate that the knowledge that underlies their practice is wider and deeper than they currently believe; to show how and why an understanding of this is vital for raising the quality of surgical education; and to offer ways of exploring these ideas with learning surgeons.

Our intention will be evident from the major focus of this chapter, which is on practice knowledge, a phenomenon well recognized in philosophy, and which is already widely discussed by health care professionals outside medicine. Indeed, in attempting to illuminate this concept we shall draw upon the extensive literature already available in the health care community and with which one of the authors of this book has been involved (see, for example, Higgs, Andressen and Fish, 2004; and Higgs, Fish and Rothwell, 2004).

We would argue that there are four main reasons why practitioners need a working understanding of practice knowledge. They need it in order to:

1. understand the knowledge that drives their decisions and actions (and to have available the language and the concepts endemic to this for the purposes of teaching, learning and assessment);

2. explain the basis of them to patients, (whose own medical knowledge has expanded exponentially as a result of the internet, but who do not have either the depth of understanding, or the wide range of other knowledge which characterizes a medical/surgical practitioner);

3. discuss them with colleagues and members of the wider health care community;

4. learn from this understanding and develop their practice.

They also need it because the nature of knowledge drawn upon and generated within the practice setting is complex in the following ways.

- ❐ It is always incomplete.
- ❐ It evolves during the collaborative relationship with colleagues and clients.
- ❐ It works with, not on, clients.
- ❐ It involves professional judgement which opens professionals up to taking risks and thus to risk being wrong.
- ❐ It is characterized by mystery at its heart.
- ❐ It is based more upon uncertainty than upon total expertise.
- ❐ It involves a spiritual dimension.
- ❐ It opens professionals up to moral answerability.
- ❐ It involves theorizing about practice *during* practice.
- ❐ It is about creating new understandings *during* practice.
- ❐ It espouses a moral and ethical approach to practice and demands from practitioners an endless critical examination of their beliefs.
- ❐ It is more dependent on artistry than on science.

Further, although the public would like to believe that professional practice is about expertise, unshakeable knowledge, and an utterly dependable technical rational base, in fact it is uncertain, messy, unique, unpredictable, unknown and the best we can have is 'wise judgement under conditions of considerable uncertainty' (Eraut, 1994, p. 17).

Clarity about what we mean by knowledge is important. Wherever understanding is missing, false assumption and unsubstantiated belief are free to roam. Our unquestioned ways of valuing knowledge can lead us to views about its nature that may cause us to mislead those we teach, and that when investigated will certainly prove untenable.

For example, in Western thought generally, society readily gives recognition and rewards to experts in factual knowledge, and tends to refer to those whose expertise involves extensive practical activity, as artisans and blue-collar workers. Although this assumption that 'doing' is more lowly than 'knowing' is prevalent, we cannot defend it through recourse to evidence from the nature of knowledge itself, but only by reference to how, as a society, we value these things. (In other societies and at other times, knowledge might be valued differently.) Indeed, the dichotomy we impose upon knowledge in this view is a false and unsustainable one. For example, doing is rarely a mindless activity (whether or not we can readily trace the knowledge that lies under it). Worse, it has led to a commonly-held but very naïve and uninformed view that an absolute gap exists between theory and practice.

Surgeons too have traditionally thought of knowledge in these narrow terms, believing (without perhaps having examined this belief in detail), that excellence in medical factual knowledge is the sole foundation of good surgical practice. This view still both reinforces and has been reinforced by the Colleges' examination system, which sets excellence in factual medical knowledge as the gold standard, and which gives far less emphasis to examining surgical practice and indeed, does not do so in the real clinical setting where the learning surgeon works and has clinical responsibility.

However, although no one would deny the importance of medical knowledge, careful thought about what happens to this factual knowledge in surgical practice (where some of it is irrelevant and none of it can be applied without adaptation to the specific context), will quickly undermine the idea that the chief component of a surgeon's expertise lies in the facts s/he learnt in order to pass a theory examination.

Given that their professional body values knowledge in this way, it is not surprising that senior surgeons often caricature themselves as 'mere carpenters' or 'only doers', and so underplay their expertise in the range of knowledge that is endemic to their practice, and which they call upon (often subconsciously) during their clinical thinking. It is likely that such attitudes are further reinforced by the tacit nature of much of practice knowledge, which makes it difficult to locate and to surface, and particularly to assess. In giving credence to this attitude, they erroneously call into question the quality of their practice by denigrating their knowledge base and denying the intelligence of their actions.

It is important to explore this further. There are far more ways of knowing, than knowing about facts and knowing how to do something. The implications of this for surgical educators are very serious. Failure by surgeons to recognize the existence of other kinds of knowledge than these two, will mean that they will continue to know more than they can ever attempt to articulate, and so will short change those for whom they have an educational responsibility. Surgeons need to recognize in principle the range of knowledge endemic to their professional practice, to analyze that which informs their own practice, to try to surface as much as possible of what lies under it, and then share it, discuss it and develop their teaching of it. It should be noted, however, that much of it cannot be taught didactically, and that teachers will therefore need to develop more explicitly than before, ways of nurturing learners as they recognize it in, and acquire it through, practice.

Key questions, then, for surgical teachers and learners are: What kinds of knowledge provide the basis of professional expertise generally? What is the knowledge base for surgery? What are the sources of practice knowledge in surgery? How can learning surgeons explore and develop them?

New perspectives on knowledge, and the nature of practice knowledge

Not knowing what one does not know

By citing the ideas of Ann Kerwin (whom he does not reference), Cox offers us six areas of ignorance to which we are all susceptible. They are shown in Table 9:1.

Table 9:1 Six areas of not knowing (see, Cox, 1999, p. 229).

Unknown unknowns	All the things we do not realize that we do not know
Known unknowns	All the things we realize that we do not know
Tacit knowledge	All the things we do not realize that we know
Error	All the things we think we know but don't
Forbidden knowledge	All taboos
Denial	Things too painful to know, which we suppress

We have presented them in a different order and format than did Cox, and have also grouped them, which he did not.

It may seem strange to begin a chapter on knowledge with this typology of not knowing, but on the other hand, recognition of ignorance is the beginning of wisdom. We offer this chapter to help surgeons, in respect of their awareness of practice knowledge, to move down the top three of this list (which we have deliberately separated from the bottom three, believing them to be of a different nature). Indeed, we hope to turn 'not knowing' to 'knowledge about', and ultimately to 'understanding'.

It is our contention that in respect of medical facts, surgeons certainly know about them, know them, and know ways of learning about them (that is, they become expert in knowing facts, otherwise known as: 'knowing that'). They also consciously acquire during their practice, the knowledge of how to enact processes and perform procedures (they become experts in doing, otherwise known as: 'knowing how'), but many neither know, nor have they recognized, the need to consider any other ways of seeing knowledge.

Re-orienting our view of knowledge

As we have already pointed out, the most common way of conceiving of knowledge for professional practice, is to think of it as divided, fairly simply, between theory and practice (or 'knowing that', and 'knowing how'; or knowing and doing). This view is so endemic to our ways of thinking about our work as professionals, that the questioning of it is a shock.

Yet, when we grapple seriously with structuring education for the professions (or within professional practice), we quickly see the following.

1. The division between theory and practice is not a watertight one (we learn the facts in order that they inform our doing; our doing is rarely mindless; and our intelligent action is one thing (acting intelligently) and not two (being intelligent on the one hand and acting on the other).

2. There needs to be interaction between theory and practice (nowadays in undergraduate professional education we intersperse blocks of time in the university setting with blocks in the practice setting so that each will enlighten the other, and at postgraduate level we oscillate between an emphasis on each).

3. That interaction (relationship) between theory and practice, however, is not an applicatory one where theory is directly and rigidly 'put into practice'. We do not, in any professional practice, impose impersonal factual knowledge onto a specific case, but rather we use and adapt (even re-interpret and re-create) that knowledge to meet the specific context and needs of the client as a person. Our professional factual knowledge is not a simple template that we impose upon the practice we meet, or through which we observe and understand it.

4. Professional practice draws on a much wider range of ways of knowing than textbook facts on the one hand and 'know-how' on the other. For example, practitioners improvise, develop insight, gain and develop knowledge through their senses (looking, touching, hearing, smelling), and they develop a repertoire of experiential knowledge, which they probably draw on most frequently of all.

5. Although in the traditional phrase 'theory and practice', theory is placed first, there are actually arguments for the 'primacy of practice' (putting practice first in this phrase or recognizing that theories emerge from practice or are created to explain, explore or extend practice). The primacy of practice encapsulates the belief that in the development of knowledge, practice comes first, and theory is developed from it.)

6. Understanding the nature of knowledge involves adopting a position about how knowledge is created. Embedded in the idea that knowledge is a given, objective, impersonal truth which is handed down by tradition, are assumptions and beliefs springing from an entire world view (positivism), which takes for granted those versions of reality and of truthful knowledge as defined by Western science or technology. The positivistic view of the world emphasizes quantities, measurements and technical

responses as solutions to all perceived problems. Critics point out that this wrongly accentuates objective versions of reality and of knowledge, and downgrades much that is most meaningful and equally of value in the world, but which is not so visible or measurable. Once we question this traditional positivistic view of knowledge, however, we find that there are other ways of seeing it - namely as socially constructed and created by practitioners. We also come to realize that all statements about the nature of the world and the nature of knowledge are fiercely contested (see Golby and Parrott, 1999; and White and Stancombe 2003, for further discussions of this).

We shall pursue this last point briefly by looking at other ways of seeing and dividing up knowledge as a whole, before turning to the detail of practice knowledge itself.

Other ways of construing the divisions of knowledge

Beneath the notion that knowledge is simply made up of theory and practice, lies the notion of knowledge as 'given', and as arriving inevitably with a particular character. If we adopt a different position, and see knowledge as created by people, as something we need to seek, and as something that can lie beneath our practice without our being aware of it, then we begin to shape a very different view. Then we see knowledge as dynamic, context bound, and made up of different ways of knowing.

One way of demonstrating this is to look at the different ways it is possible to divide up knowledge, and how, within that, different disciplines use 'proof' and 'truth' differently, and see the world from different angles. Indeed, each of us needs to be aware of our own position with respect to this, since our own education will have emphasized one way of conceiving of knowledge, which we may never have challenged.

'Education within a discipline stamps us with particular views about the origins of knowledge, ways of seeing truth, what counts as evidence (ways of handling proof), views about theory and practice, and views about appropriate means of achieving rigour. Even the very meaning of rigour itself is disciplinarily-determined. It is easy when one is steeped in a particular way of seeing knowledge, to apply that approach unthinkingly to other kinds of knowledge (such as knowledge of another field) where it may not be appropriate or applicable.'

(Higgs, Andressen and Fish, 2004, p. 64.)

The work of Phenix (1964) helps us to think about ways of seeing knowledge as a whole. He defines six 'Realms of Meaning': Symbolics (language and mathematics); Empirics (the sciences of the physical world, of living things and of humans); Esthetics [sic] (the arts); Synnoetics [sic] (personal knowledge); Ethics (moral knowledge) and Synoptics (history, religion, philosophy). In a not dissimilar model, Carper, in nursing, identified four fundamental patterns of knowing: Empirics (science); Aesthetics (art); Personal knowledge; and Ethics (moral knowledge); and proposed that none of them alone should be considered sufficient or mutually exclusive for work in nursing (see Carper, 1978). Building on Carper's work, Sarter added a fifth way of knowing called 'intellectual/interpretive', which includes gaining knowledge through philosophical analysis, metaphysical analysis or hermeneutics.

Probably the best way to illustrate the key differences between disciplines is to consider the arts and sciences as follows.

Ways of knowing in the arts and sciences

Of course it is true that the fields of art and science are by no means mutually exclusive, since it is possible to find deep aesthetic meanings in things studied scientifically, and to find scientific truth in aesthetic experiences, but the key difference between them is in the kinds of understanding gained and the contrasting views of the world to which they give rise.

Scientists come to know empirical truth via observation and experimentation, which is then generalized. Knowledge in science is expressed in general laws and theories, connected with observable particulars by way of prediction and verification. Science strives for objective certainties and often downplays the theoretical nature of its discoveries. Scientists see these certainties as new truths and expect others to apply them to practice. Being caught up unconsciously into this view of knowledge, and being wrongly persuaded that this is the only (right) way of construing the world, can drive one to expect to be able, *in all fields* to source knowledge, to verify it, to hold an applicatory view of the relationship between theory and practice, and to work with rigour to drive for objective certainties, and prove their truths. It is this view, when brought into professional practice (where knowledge is eternally incomplete and insufficient) that causes unrealistic expectations e.g. that objective knowledge of all aspects of practice exists somewhere in the universe waiting to be discovered.

By comparison, ways of knowing in the arts offer other perspectives on professional practice. The arts, Phenix says, are crucially concerned with 'particularity'. Thus, aesthetic understanding is not contained in propositions but in particular and presented objects (like poems, pictures, plays, novels, symphonies). Such objects may contain propositions and truths (like those found in love poetry or in the plays we call tragedies), but the truth of the propositions offered in such literature, is not alone the measure of the meaning of it as a work of art. The language of art (unlike science) is non-discursive, symbolical and metaphorical. The logic of art is that of language or music or the visual arts, not of mathematics. Further, artists theorize in practice, as part of their practice (see Phenix, 1964, p.154). The quality of a work of art depends on the quality of the manner in which the materials are organized into a patterned whole to become an organic unity whose form underpins its content. The value of a piece of art comes then, from an examination of its form and content and their inter-relation. Evidence must relate to that piece of art and refer only generally to aesthetic principles. The truth embodied in a piece of art is subtle, is validated by the *frisson of recognition* created in the audience, and is often deeper and more enduring than that proposed in scientific laws. (The truths embodied in Shakespeare's plays and sonnets speak equally to people of the 21st Century, where many of the truths of his scientific contemporaries have long since been disproved and discarded.) This of course is not to deny that some scientific truths too have demonstrated considerable endurance.

Ways of knowing in professional practice

Once it is recognized that knowledge can be seen differently in the sciences compared with the arts, it becomes clear that for the professional practitioner, too, there are particular ways of understanding and construing knowledge, which will open up new ways of seeing and thinking about practice. This sub-section seeks to explore a range of ways of thinking about knowledge from a professional practitioner's standpoint.

Practice, theory and the primacy of practice

There are many who argue that there is no hierarchical order between theory and practice, but that they are more intimately related than the phrase suggests. Some characterize theory and practice as coexisting and combining in practice settings. Some talk about a dialectical relationship (Higgs and Titchen, 2001), which confronts the differences between knowing and doing and reconciles these differences, thus producing a higher order process of doing-knowing, which encompasses them both. Harnessing the combined power of knowing and doing is often invaluable in dealing with the contradictions, uncertainties and complexities of practice.

Others, however, as we have said above, argue that it is practice which actually comes first in the creation of new knowledge. This idea is traditionally referred to in the phrase the primacy of practice. It is Gilbert Ryle who called our attention to the arguments for the primacy of practice. In his seminal book on the philosophy of mind, *The Concept of Mind*, he challenged the traditional relationship, by declaring:

'Efficient practice precedes the theory of it … It is … possible for people intelligently to perform some sorts of operations when they are not yet able to consider any propositions enjoining how they should be performed.'

He added:

'Some intelligent performances are not controlled by any interior acknowledgments of the principles applied to them.'

(Ryle, 1949, p. 31)

and:

'… we learn how by practice, schooled indeed by criticism and example, but often quite unaided by any lessons in the theory.'

(Ryle, 1949, p. 41)

It should of course be noted here that he is not saying that there is no knowledge underlying such actions, but rather that the knowing is in the doing, that is, that the (factual) knowledge used often lies beneath our consciousness, and is a part of the action rather than separable from it. This must mean that some factual knowledge is learnt in and during practice, not before it.

Ryle contextualized his argument by debunking what he famously characterized as 'the myth of the mind' as a 'ghost in the machine' of the body'. This was an idea bequeathed by Plato via Descartes to the 20th Century and which is unthinkingly perpetuated in many of the bodily metaphors we employ even today for referring to the mind. Ryle contended that we should not imagine that behind intelligent action is the ghost of intelligent thought. Instead, he argued:

'... when I do something intelligently, i.e. thinking what I am doing, I am doing one thing and not two. My performance has a special procedure or manner, not special antecedents.'

(Ryle 1949, p. 32).

He also made the point that theorizing is a practice itself, and offered us the useful term 'intelligent practice':

'... intelligent practice is not a step-child of theory. On the contrary, theorizing is one practice amongst others and is itself intelligently or stupidly conducted.'

(Ryle, 1949, p. 27).

Practice knowledge and practice epistemology

We have been arguing then, that underlying and implicit in practice in all professions is a whole range of knowledge which is special to practice and practitioners, (often referred to as practice knowledge), and that it is important for practitioners to understand its nature.

The branch of philosophy that investigates the nature of knowledge generally (its origins, methods, and limits) is known as epistemology. Practice epistemology, therefore, is the technical and shorthand term for referring to 'the nature of knowledge and the processes of generation of knowledge, which underlie practice' (Richardson, Higgs and Abrandt Dahlgren, 2004, p. 5). Practitioners who have a working knowledge of practice epistemology understand what drives their decisions and actions, are able to explain the basis of them to patients, colleagues and members of the wider health care community, and 'recognize how they can learn from this understanding and develop their practice' and its knowledge base (ibid).

The creation of practice knowledge

It is, of course, also the responsibility of each profession to explicate and generate professional knowledge which is appropriate to contemporary practice (that is, each profession must develop its practice knowledge base, which is inevitably dynamic). To do so requires an understanding of what is involved in practice knowledge. How this is seen (as we have shown) is affected by our conscious and unconscious beliefs and values.

We would argue that both the conduct of professional practice and the evolution of professional knowledge involves creating knowledge *in practice*. This also means that practitioners are the source of practice knowledge. Practice knowledge is the outcome of reflection by individuals and professional groups on their knowledge and practice. Formal practice knowledge is that which has been further critiqued and sharpened by publication and public debate.

It will be noted in the following discussion, that knowledge that is generated in practice, during practice, is in fact a major component of practice knowledge.

The components of practice knowledge

It will be evident by now that there is no one correct way to characterize the make-up of practice knowledge. How we see it will be determined by our particular world views, which will result in our emphasizing particular components (perhaps at the expense of others). Accordingly, we offer two formal views of the components of practice knowledge (that is, views already available in the literature), together with our own, more detailed way of seeing this. We also call attention to the nature of practice knowledge as tacit, implicit or explicit. We then summarize all three views of knowledge in Table 9:2, and offer, in Figure 9:1, our own detailed map of practice knowledge for professionals, and invite readers' critique and consideration of it.

Our intention in all this is both to alert surgeons to this important debate (since teachers' and learners' assumptions about knowledge will affect how they discuss their practice), and to make a contribution to that debate.

A range of views about the components of practice knowledge

As we have seen, the most fundamental division of knowledge is into theory and practice. Where practice knowledge is seen as divided thus, the terms used are: 'propositional knowledge' (for theoretical or formal factual knowledge), and 'procedural knowledge' (for knowing how to do things) (see Ryle, 1949). Most of those who write about knowledge in relation to professional practice use these two basic terms. Higgs and Titchen, (2001), offer three main divisions, in effect recognizing one component for propositional knowledge and two for procedural knowledge. They thus see knowledge as follows: knowledge derived from research and formal theory; knowledge derived from professional experience; and knowledge derived from personal experience. Eraut, (2001), by contrast, emphasizes the formal and personal aspects. He sees propositional knowledge as one key component (but extends its meaning by offering 'codified knowledge' as a better term for what he sees as 'knowledge that includes propositions (including propositions about skills)' and also as 'public knowledge which is controlled by editors, peer review, and debate and given status by being incorporated into educational programmes'. He uses the term 'personal knowledge' to mean 'the cognitive resource which a person brings to a situation that enables them to think and perform'. He argues that this incorporates codified knowledge in a personalized form, together with procedural knowledge (including skills) and process knowledge (which he does not explain further), experiential knowledge and impressions in episodic memory' (Eraut, 2001, p.114).

Our view of the key aspects of practice knowledge

We have tried to look at professional practice overall, without first imposing on it any clear-cut categories, and as a result would suggest that in fact there seem to be at least fourteen aspects of knowledge that shape practice. Many of these do not comfortably fit even the basic categories of Ryle's original dichotomy. For example, we would place in propositional knowledge many more elements of factual knowledge, not all of which are public in quite the way Eraut describes, and whilst we acknowledge the procedural elements as the main ones (believing in the primacy of practice), we see many elements of knowledge in practice as partly theoretical and partly practical.

We believe these key components to be: knowledge of facts of all kinds (propositional knowledge); knowledge of up-to-date medical thought and research (evidence-based knowledge); knowing how to act and how to get things done (procedural knowledge); knowing how to organize and adapt propositional knowledge to the context (propositional adaptation knowledge); knowing how to improvise procedural knowledge to suit the given case (procedural improvisation knowledge); knowledge of the traditions of the profession and conduct of its members (professional knowledge); knowledge gained through the sense of touch, sound, smell, and sight (sensory knowledge); knowledge of ethical and moral principles of practice which guides safe adaptation and improvisation (ethical knowledge); knowledge gained as a result of previous experience and reflection upon it (experiential knowledge); knowledge created during practice (practice-generated knowledge); knowledge of the higher levels of thought that shape the creation, adaptation and development of practice knowledge, and the overall processes of clinical thinking (meta-cognitive knowledge); knowledge for which there is no immediate explanation (intuitive knowledge); knowledge which comes suddenly as a fully-fledged vision, without the underlying reasoning being apparent (insight/imagination); knowledge of one's own strengths, weaknesses and limitations (self-knowledge).

Of course, we would want to see all this knowledge coming together ultimately in the fluent and holistic practice of an expert practitioner, but we believe that better knowledge of the components provides a vocabulary in which to discuss the details, and a means of diagnosing problems or particular expertise in any of them.

Tacit, implicit and explicit knowledge

As we show in Table 9:2, we believe a remarkable amount of this practice knowledge to be tacit or at best implicit. Indeed, as the table shows, we see only one of the fourteen elements that make up practice as entirely explicit.

By 'tacit knowledge' we mean that knowledge which we do not even recognize that we have. This may be because it is buried inside our thinking and doing, and beneath our experiences and expertise, to a level that renders it unable readily to be retrieved and made conscious; or (in some cases) it may be that it is actually by its very nature ineffable (inexpressible, unable to be described and characterized).

Much of such knowledge may always have been (and some will continue to be) tacit in our professional practice, or it may once have been implicit or even explicit, but we no longer see it because routine and custom have put us on auto-pilot, or simply got in the way of our recognizing it. This, of course, is a great problem for the education of less experienced practitioners. By definition, much of that knowledge which is tacit in senior doctors and surgeons, is the bedrock of good professional practice and wherever possible needs to be opened up to learners (for reasons explained above), which means that their teachers must struggle to bring back to consciousness as much of it as possible. Indeed, learners need to seek it actively from their seniors in order to lay the foundations for their own practice.

By comparison, 'implicit knowledge' lies just under the surface of the practices of professionals, or can be seen as lying within products, procedures, processes and organizations. Compared with tacit knowledge, it is much more possible to surface implicit knowledge, embedded as it is within services, structures, methods and techniques. It is true that some professionals who are now teachers may themselves, in the past, have merely been trained in or socialized in handling processes and procedures, and thus have learnt to enact them without unpacking such implicit knowledge and understanding. This will make it more difficult for them to share their implicit knowledge with their learners, but it is now imperative that they work to do so, in order to promote the critique and discussion currently needed to prepare professionals to explain and defend their knowledge-in-use amongst colleagues and patients, and in public and even courts of law.

Other important forms of implicit knowledge are more personal, and relate to matters like beliefs, assumptions, values, and personal theories. To an extent this is about beliefs rather than knowledge, but there is a relationship between these two. Implicit knowledge of this kind can mostly be made explicit with time and thought, but only once its significance has been realized. Again, both teacher and learner need to attend to 'surfacing or re-surfacing' the implicit. This is not only easier than unearthing or reifying tacit knowledge, it is even possible that the learner can achieve some of this by inference and without the help of the teacher. However, both teacher and learner need to work at this.

'Explicit knowledge' is of course that which is publicly documented and structured, or as Eraut calls it 'codified', or that which a practitioner can state clearly. This can include facts, methods, interpretations, conclusions and reports about best practice. It is of course easily demonstrable how much knowledge is actually explicit and in the public arena. In many health care professions, in order to enhance their status, a premium has been set on explicating as much of this as possible (especially in relation to good practice in the profession and in the education for that profession). Surgical examples would include text books about medical knowledge, practical processes, and operative procedures as well as writing like that of Gawande, (2001), and reports of research. It is interesting to note that there is as yet little literature which shares publicly good practice in surgical *education*.

While some practice knowledge will always remain tacit, we believe that much of what is currently implicit in professional practice could be made explicit. We believe that making as much as possible explicit would seriously improve the rigour of teaching professional processes and procedures. Careful reflection on practice and enquiry into it will yield the secret of much of its underlying knowledge, and working with this to turn it into understanding will show us new ways to develop our practice.

Table 9:2 A summary of ways of seeing practice knowledge.

Source	Components
Ryle 1949	Propositional knowledge (which informs practice) Procedural knowledge (which is about action and the knowledge within it of how to do it)
Higgs, *et al*, 2001	Knowledge derived from research and formal theory (propositional knowledge) Knowledge derived from professional experience (craft knowledge) Knowledge derived from personal experience (experiential knowledge)

Eraut 2000	Codified knowledge (public knowledge which is controlled by editors, etc, and given status by being incorporated into education)
	 (Includes propositions about skilled behaviour, but not skills or knowing how)
	 Is explicit
	
	 Personal knowledge (the cognitive resource which a person brings to a situation that enables them to think and perform). This incorporates:
	
	     codified knowledge in a personalized form
	     procedural knowledge (including skills)
	     process knowledge
	     experiential knowledge
	     impressions in episodic memory
	
	 May be implicit or tacit

Our own view	Propositional knowledge (most explicit, some implicit) Evidence-based knowledge (explicit) Propositional adaptation knowledge (not currently explicit) Procedural knowledge (much of it tacit or implicit) Procedural improvisation knowledge (not currently explicit) Professional knowledge (part explicit, part implicit) Sensory knowledge (much of it tacit) Ethical knowledge (some explicit, some implicit) Experiential knowledge (implicit, unless reflected upon) Practice-generated knowledge (mostly tacit) Meta-cognitive knowledge (mostly tacit or implicit) Intuitive knowledge (explicit or implicit) Insight/imagination (mostly tacit) Self-knowledge (partly explicit, partly implicit, partly tacit)

Affected and shaped by values, and always context specific to the clinical setting

PROCEDURAL KNOWLEDGE

Skills, know-how, processes, procedures (related to: clinical; managerial; educational; research; organizational; Trust-level)

PROPOSITIONAL KNOWLEDGE

Formal specialist theory, formal generic theory, knowledge of context, of education, of management, of organization, of profession, of society

PROCEDURAL IMPROVISATION KNOWLEDGE

How to use and adapt know-how safely to the given context

EVIDENCE-BASED KNOWLEDGE

Knowledge of all appropriate research where relevant

PROPOSITIONAL ADAPTATION KNOWLEDGE

Knowing how to reorganize factual knowledge/skills to respond to the given case

METACOGNITIVE KNOWLEDGE

Knowledge of the structure of knowledge and higher-order ways of organizing knowing

PROFESSIONAL KNOWLEDGE AND CONDUCT

Knowledge of the traditions and parameters of the practice of the profession and its legal framework

EXPERIENTIAL KNOWLEDGE

Knowledge gained from undergoing experiences and reflecting on them to make sense of them and learn from them

PRACTICE-GENERATED KNOWLEDGE

New knowledge created through undertaking, exploring, and theorizing an aspect of professional practice (can lead to new propositional and procedural knowledge)

ETHICAL KNOWLEDGE

Knowledge of ethical and moral principles that guide all professional practice and that will shape the safe improvisation of procedural knowledge and the re-organization of propositional knowledge

SENSORY KNOWLEDGE

All that knowledge, both procedural and propositional, that comes to the practitioner through the senses

SELF-KNOWLEDGE

Accurate knowledge of own personal characteristics, values and beliefs, plus procedural capabilities and grasp of propositional knowledge

INTUITIVE KNOWLEDGE

Something that we know or are moved to do but cannot (yet) give logical or evidential grounds for

INSIGHT/IMAGINATION

A sudden holistic grasp of an aspect of procedural, propositional or self-knowledge, or knowledge of others

Figure 9:1 A map of practice knowledge for professionals generally.

Mapping practice knowledge for professionals generally

In the map (Figure 9:1), we have added more detail within each of these areas, in terms of both the content of components and their relationship. It will, for example, be noted that the two main divisions of theory and practice are where we begin, but that much of the rest of this knowledge, being both theoretical and practical (as befits the complex inter-relationship of theory and practice), is represented as both propositional and procedural. We have demonstrated this both in the layout of the map and in the shading used. It will also be evident that we have honoured the primacy of practice by placing procedural knowledge first. The small print in each component attempts to give some examples of the kinds of knowledge we are referring to. We have used a standard size for all boxes except that for knowledge generated in practice, because that is the component we believe to be most significant, but we do not wish to imply comparisons between any of the rest.

The practice knowledge of surgeons and how to teach and assess it

This section will translate what we have said about practice knowledge for professionals generally into that which is specific to surgical practice. In particular, it will characterize the kinds of knowledge that surgeons use in practice, and will first look at the sources of practice knowledge available for learning surgeons to access.

The sources of practice knowledge for surgeons

Traditionally the key sources of knowledge for the learning surgeon were considered to be the consultant for whom they worked and the text books from which they learnt medical theoretical knowledge, and learnt about technical and procedural knowledge. Once the wider range of knowledge drawn upon in professional practice is recognized however, a commensurately wider set of sources emerge from which to learn that knowledge.

Cox draws our attention to the fact that:

'... clinicians 'think on their feet' during a consultation as they consider what to do next ....
Some clinicians can think aloud as they work, offering trainees a running account of what they are looking at, what they are looking for and what they have found. Surgeons may explain the steps, and the surgical anatomy and pathology, as they work through an operation. But, observably, most clinicians do not. This thinking while working is usually brought out for comment only after the consultation is over, if at all.'

(Cox, 1999, p. 272)

As a reminder to teacher and learner alike, we have attempted to list the wider sources of practice knowledge for surgeons in Table 9:3. It will be noted that we value the service

Table 9:3 The sources of practice knowledge for surgeons.

Service commitment	Engaging in professional practice in theatre, ward and clinic, but doing so mindfully, so as to be aware of at least some of its components
	Improvising procedural knowledge
	Adapting propositional knowledge
	Creating new knowledge during practice
	Professionals as models of various kinds
Practising procedures	Repeating procedures and processes, but reflectively, so that this is not mindless repetition of practice irrespective of quality
Reflection	Analyzing critically actions, thoughts and knowledge embedded in practice, particularly in relation to own practice and experience
Those outside the service commitment	Written knowledge: books, journals, research papers, internet
	Oral: lectures, talks
	Demonstration
	Master classes
	Dictats from government and national and local organizations
Personal interaction	Learner asking probing questions and using talk to clarify understanding
	Engaging in professional conversations
	Induction into the traditions of practice enshrined in professional conduct of senior colleagues by discussion with them
	Discussion with the inter-professional team in theatre, clinic, ward
Self	Experiential, personal and professional experiences reflected upon
	Sensory (observation and tactile, auditory and olfactory senses)
	Memories of experiences and patterns
	Intuition
	Insight
History and narrative	Anecdotes of earlier cases
	Making a narrative of an episode of practice and enriching it with the help of reflection, and of others who were there
Education	Being taught
	Being supervised
	Using own educational portfolio
	Observing practice
	Engaging in practice together with reflection
	Being assessed
	Learning to self-assess

commitment as a major source of knowledge, that we have placed the practical elements first, and coupled them with reflection, and that we have highlighted the importance of the multi-professional (or disciplinary) team in theatre, ward and clinic and of the learner interacting with colleagues in order to clarify understanding. We also acknowledge the importance of narrative (both of immediate events and the history of other relevant cases), by means of which the consultant can extend the passive knowledge of the learner.

Mapping the components of knowledge that surgeons use in practice

Given this overview of sources of practice knowledge and the overall map of professional knowledge generally, we can now turn to the details of surgeons' practice knowledge. In Figure 9:2, we have taken the headings as offered in Figure 9:1, and offered in small print the surgical examples and versions of these. It will be noted that we believe that how teacher and learners see all this and accord it significance will be determined by their values. How it can be adapted and used by learners and teachers in practice will be shaped by the given clinical context.

In Figure 9:2, again, we have enlarged the box relating to the generation of practice knowledge because we believe that this aspect of knowledge is currently underplayed by learning surgeons. This is perhaps because of the (groundless) fear that the public would see this as a licence for reckless and undisciplined surgical practice, when in fact, out of every individual surgical case there is likely to emerge some new knowledge for the given learner (otherwise how does their surgical practice develop?).

How surgeons use knowledge differently at different learning stages

We pointed out in Chapter 7, in respect of clinical thinking, that medical school students learn and engage in fairly rigid scientific processes of diagnostic thinking, and that only postgraduate doctors can learn the subtleties of deliberation in the practice setting. Eraut points out that there is evolution of both knowledge structure and diagnostic skill as the postgraduate becomes more experienced. What is more, he implies that in postgraduate medical practice, learning new ways of structuring the knowledge already possessed takes precedence over accruing large amounts of new propositional knowledge. He states, for example, that increase in knowledge of pathophysiology is small compared with the organization of that knowledge to make it more readily and rapidly available (see Eraut and du Boulay, 2000). They acknowledge that the work of Chang *et al*, (1998), had emphasized this previously. Quoting Grant and Marsden, (1988), Eraut and du Boulay remind us that every practitioner's knowledge base is highly individual and will have evolved from their previous personal clinical experience. The knowledge of novices is largely scientific in nature and has been structured for them by its presentation in text books, and lectures which highlight the intrinsic structure of the academic discipline. Few teachers in medical school invite learners to re-structure this for themselves (make it their own). Postgraduates gradually have to find their own way of re-packaging their knowledge to enable it to be drawn on quickly and appropriately in their everyday clinical

Affected and shaped by values, and always context specific to the clinical setting

PROCEDURAL KNOWLEDGE

Clinical thinking, clinical processes, technical and operative procedures, educational processes, managerial processes

PROPOSITIONAL KNOWLEDGE

Generic medical and surgical knowledge, specialist medical and surgical knowledge, profession-wide knowledge, knowledge of organizations and social knowledge of Trust requirements

PROCEDURAL IMPROVISATION KNOWLEDGE

How to use, and adapt clinical processes and technical and operative procedures safely to the given context

EVIDENCE-BASED KNOWLEDGE

Knowledge of all appropriate research

PROPOSITIONAL ADAPTATION KNOWLEDGE

Knowing how to reorganize factual medical/surgical knowledge/skills in response to a given case

METACOGNITIVE KNOWLEDGE

Knowledge of the structure of medical and surgical knowledge, and of ways of charting clinical thinking and of how to reflect

PROFESSIONAL KNOWLEDGE AND CONDUCT

The values and standards of the Surgical Royal Colleges and the medico-legal boundaries. Professional conduct and values in clinical settings

CASE KNOWLEDGE AND OTHER EXPERIENTIAL KNOWLEDGE

Relevant personal experience; propositional and procedural knowledge gained from own experience in theatre, ward and clinic and the sense made of this through personal reflection

PRACTICE-GENERATED KNOWLEDGE

Knowledge of how to theorize practice, and of how to investigate practice; the creation by learners of new responses to challenges they meet in the clinical setting; the emergence of professional judgement; the development of surgical expertise (new know-how); the creation of whole new ways of treating surgical disease. All of this, using SAFE improvisation

ETHICAL KNOWLEDGE

Knowledge of ethical and moral principles that guide medical and surgical practice and that will shape the safe improvisation of procedural knowledge and the re-organization of propositional knowledge

SENSORY KNOWLEDGE

All that medical and surgical knowledge, both procedural and propositional, that comes to the practitioner through the senses

SELF-KNOWLEDGE

Accurate knowledge of own personal characteristics, values and beliefs, and of own procedural capabilities in medicine and surgery and grasp of propositional knowledge

INTUITIVE KNOWLEDGE

Clinical thought, and taking clinical action without objective evidence to support it, but which is then seen to be appropriate

INSIGHT/IMAGINATION

A sudden holistic grasp of an aspect of procedural or propositional medical or surgical knowledge, or self-knowledge, or an ability to put oneself into the mind of another

Figure 9:2 A map of practice knowledge for surgeons.

practice. Schmidt and Boshuinzen, (1993) set out a model for considering the difference between novices and experts and their use of knowledge. They say that being an expert is not knowing more than novices but merely organizing knowledge differently, combining it with increasing experience of cases, until the cases become more significant than the scientific knowledge. Surgeon educators need crucially to know where their learner is with respect to this, in order to help them to develop further.

To explore this understanding with the learner, the teacher will need to ask the learner to talk through the knowledge and experience drawn on in relation first to the theoretical pathways 7:3, 7:4, and 7:5 above, and then in relation to a given case on these pathways. See the following section.

In all this it should be remembered that 'expertise lies not in the knowledge *per se*, but in the judgement of what's pertinent and important' (Cox, 1999, p. 277).

Focusing on the knowledge used in clinical thinking

'The theory-practice relationship is shaped by the 'tacit resources' that consultant surgeons continuously develop in their practice. SHOs and Surgeon Educators will benefit from surgeons' revelation of tacit values, beliefs, attitudes, assumptions, expectations, feelings, knowledge and experience.'

(Brigley, *et al*, 2003)

In Chapter 7 we talked about the surgeon's thinking processes. In this chapter we are focusing on the knowledge that fuels this thinking. In cases where the condition is common, where there is one obvious way of managing the surgical problem, and the patient is fit and well so that there are few if any medically confounding factors, the knowledge that fuels surgeons' thinking will mainly be procedural, propositional and evidence-based knowledge, and this will be used in a standardized and well rehearsed way. It will require little of the more sophisticated forms of knowledge, such as experiential, practice-generated, or sensory. This thinking process and the knowledge which fuels it here is that most commonly used by novices in surgical practice, and is the foundation of learning to manage successfully more complex cases.

By contrast, for example, an elderly patient with many co-morbid medical conditions may have a range of treatment options which run from no active surgical intervention to complex technical and operative interventions. This will require the use of most, if not all of the knowledge described in Figure 9:2. Interestingly, the thinking processes in such a case are very likely to call upon only a small amount of propositional and straightforward procedural knowledge, and a much greater amount of many of the other forms described.

Following Eraut's ideas, we believe that our sophisticated descriptors of knowledge show more clearly than previously what influences and drives surgeons' redevelopment of knowledge and what shapes their reconfiguration of its structures for more efficient use in practice. These descriptions, we believe, will assist surgeons to understand how they think, and enable them to examine and discuss with learners the range and structure of the knowledge they are drawing upon. Those who teach in surgical practice will also find them useful, in enabling them to draw distinctions between different practitioners at different levels of personal development.

Surgeons who aspire to great expertise in the profession must develop (and more consciously than ever before) this whole range of knowledge. Surgeons who become fluent in practice will come to use this knowledge unconsciously, but will be able to articulate it where necessary. Teachers, however will need to make their use of this knowledge explicit, and learners will need to incorporate their awareness of these matters into their clinical thinking. This can best be done by talking and writing reflectively about clinical cases with the intention of identifying the knowledge components drawn upon, in ways we exemplify below in relation to the three scenarios which we first used in Chapter 7.

The scenario of a new outpatient consultation

The context of the case

A female secondary school teacher of forty-eight years is sent to the surgical clinic by her GP, asking for an opinion as to the cause and treatment of her abdominal pain. She has suffered three attacks of pain and on one occasion required admission to hospital whilst on holiday in Spain. Gallstones were identified on ultrasound examination. She is now seeking advice on preventing further attacks of what the GP has diagnosed as biliary colic. She is sent an outpatient appointment in February.

Framing the problem

She is seen in the new outpatient clinic by the SpR who:

- extracts the salient features from the GP letter **(propositional medical knowledge, experiential knowledge)**;
- begins to think about the possible diagnosis … **(propositional adaptation knowledge)**
- recalls his previous experience of this condition **(experiential knowledge)**;
- as a matter of principle holds the presenting diagnosis as questionable **(propositional adaptation knowledge)**;
- has three other key possibilities in mind as to her problem (peptic ulceration, hiatus hernia, or colonic problems) **(propositional medical knowledge)**.

He thus frames the complex clinical problem as having four diagnostic possibilities which he must place in order of probability **(propositional medical knowledge)**.

The scenario of a new outpatient consultation *continued:*

The clinical reasoning process

He then attempts to make sense of the case by observing the patient **(sensory knowledge)**, taking a history **(medical procedural knowledge)** and critiquing the GP's diagnosis by recognizing pictures, patterns and signs that will allow him to order his four possibilities **(procedural knowledge, sensory knowledge, propositional knowledge, evidence-based knowledge, practice generated knowledge)**.

His observation and the patient's history reveal a fit woman with no co-morbid factors. There has been no history of jaundice. Examination is unremarkable and reveals no abdominal scars **(propositional medical knowledge, propositional adaptation knowledge, procedural knowledge)**.

The diagnosis of biliary colic is the most likely from this evidence. No further tests are deemed necessary and he advises the operation of cholecystectomy by the laparoscopic technique **(propositional knowledge, procedural knowledge, evidence-based knowledge)**. He takes consent, and prepares the required paperwork necessary to list the patient for the operation **(propositional and procedural knowledge and ethical knowledge)**. The clinical solution is thus secured.

The deliberative process

Before finishing the consultation the patient asks when the operation is likely to take place and how long will she be off work. She says that she is the Head of Department for French and that the final examinations of her students are in June. The registrar tells her that the normal waiting time is about three months and that the Trust requires patients to be treated in the order of listing **(procedural knowledge)**. She may need to be off work for between three to six weeks depending on recovery. She requests that she has the operation in the school holidays, preferably in August

The registrar brings in the consultant surgeon to seek his opinion about the patient's request **(procedural knowledge, procedural improvisation knowledge, ethical knowledge)**. The consultant talks with the patient and agrees with her to aim to book the operation in August, **(ethical knowledge, procedural improvisation knowledge, propositional knowledge of Trust and organization, propositional adaptation knowledge)** assuming that no further adverse events occur before that time **(propositional and experiential knowledge)**. In exercising this practical wisdom he has added to the conclusions reached by the SpR and taken account of the feelings and needs of the patient **(insight/imagination)**. The consultation is completed and the patient leaves. The consultant talks with the registrar and explains his reasons for making the decisions as he did **(self-knowledge)**. The agreed action plan is recorded in the patient's notes **(procedural knowledge)**.

Comment

This case is clinically straightforward but introduces the patient's perspective with respect to accepting the medical diagnosis and treatment. It will be noted that propositional and procedural medical knowledge are the main components of knowledge drawn upon in this case.

The scenario of new clinical thinking during treatment

The context of the case

A female patient is admitted for laparoscopic cholecystectomy to the day-case unit, which is separate from the main hospital and has no overnight stay beds. She is the first case of the morning and it is anticipated that she will go home in the early evening. The case will be done under general anaesthetic by an experienced SpR assisted by an SHO in surgery. The consultant is available in the theatre suite.

Framing the problem

The patient is anaesthetised, the SpR has inserted the ports and begins the dissection of the gallbladder **(procedural surgical knowledge)**. The gallbladder is very dilated with omentum stuck to it and there are some patches of necrosis in the wall **(propositional medical knowledge, practice-generated knowledge)**. The SpR expresses surprise that the case has been listed for day surgery **(practice-generated knowledge, procedural knowledge, experiential knowledge)**. He begins to mull over the problems of day-case selection for laparoscopic cholecystectomies, and wonders uneasily about the likely logistical problems that will ensue about acquiring a bed for, and transport of, the patient to the main hospital **(procedural improvisation knowledge, propositional adaptation knowledge)**. While thinking this, he proceeds carefully but after half and hour still has not identified the appropriate anatomy to be able to advance the operation **(procedural improvisation knowledge)**. He then realizes that his immediate practical complex clinical problem is to decide whether he can continue with the patient as a day case, and how long he should proceed with the minimally invasive procedure **(insight, self-knowledge, intuitive knowledge)**. He is aware of the body language and comment from others in the theatre. The consultant anaesthetist is muttering about case selection, the likely need for an overnight bed and cancelling the rest of the list **(sensory knowledge, ethical knowledge)**. The complex clinical problem here is the clinician's, not the patient's **(insight, self-knowledge)**!

The scenario of new clinical thinking during treatment *continued:*

The clinical reasoning process

The SpR works through in his mind the pros and cons of proceeding with a difficult dissection, which might cause damage to other important structures near the gallbladder **(medical propositional and procedural knowledge, experiential knowledge, self-knowledge, and ethical knowledge)**. Some of this he shares with the rest of the theatre team. He questions whether it might not be more prudent to convert the operation to an open procedure **(procedural improvisation knowledge)**. He considers the arguments logically, and calculates that there is a case for spending a modest time in further trying to display carefully the anatomy **(procedural improvisation knowledge)**. He also recognizes the disruption that will be caused by failing to do this as a day case **(professional knowledge, practice-generated knowledge, ethical knowledge)** not to mention the fact that the department may loose some face in having a second case in two weeks that could not go home on the day of surgery **(experiential knowledge)**.

The deliberative process

The SpR calls the consultant surgeon for advice, explaining that he realizes that conversion to an open procedure may be required but he has never before opened a patient listed for day surgery **(self-knowledge, ethical knowledge, procedural improvisation knowledge)**. The consultant scrubs and takes over the case. He confirms the hard stuck nature of the gallbladder and after a total of one hour of surgery makes a decision to convert the procedure to an open cholecystectomy **(self-knowledge, practice-generated knowledge, procedural improvisation knowledge)**. He directs the scrub nurse to prepare for a change in procedure and requests that things are put in motion to find an in-patient bed as well as to inform the ward medical staff about the change of plan **(propositional and procedural knowledge)**. The theatre staff find the telephone number of the patient's relatives in order that they may be informed of the decision **(procedural improvisation knowledge, ethical knowledge)**.

The consultant performs a successful open cholecystectomy and the SpR closes the wound **(procedural surgical knowledge)**. The consultant discusses the case with the SpR and SHO and prepares them for explaining things to the patient **(ethical knowledge, procedural knowledge, experiential knowledge)**. A record of the decisions and actions is made in the patient's notes **(procedural knowledge)**. As a consequence, one case on the planned list is postponed because of insufficient time to complete the list. Arrangements are put in place for someone to talk to that patient, to explain why this has happened and rebook their operation putting them first on the list at the next available time **(insight/imagination, procedural knowledge, ethical knowledge, propositional knowledge)**. The patient is finally admitted to the ward and discharged five days later after an uncomplicated recovery.

Comment

It will be noted in this case that there is considerably less call upon propositional and procedural knowledge and far greater use of a range of other knowledge components.

The scenario of the wider issues of clinical practice

The context of the case

It is the 14th of August and the ward medical staff are new. A patient is on the operating list for abdominal aortic aneurysm surgery the following morning and is waiting at home for the call to be told that there is a suitable bed available. He has already been cancelled by the Trust once because of bed problems. The critical care unit now has a patient with MRSA in her wound and five other patients have become contacts. The unit is full with respect to the number of critical care staff available to nurse the patients.

Framing the problem

MRSA is a recurring problem in the Trust **(propositional knowledge)**. There is a new Trust policy in place that the bed manager discusses the case with the Trust lead for MRSA who is a consultant microbiologist **(propositional and procedural knowledge)**. This is done and the bed manager offers a solution that arrangements could be made to 'special' the patient on the surgical ward, which is clean **(procedural improvisational knowledge)**. This is accepted. The ward medical staff are informed and the patient is phoned and advised to come into the hospital. There is a sense of relief that another cancellation of this particular patient will be avoided **(experiential knowledge, practice-generated knowledge)**. The consultant vascular surgeon finds out about this arrangement at eight o'clock on the day of surgery when he does a pre-operative visit **(practice-generated knowledge)**. His problem now is: does he accept these arrangements or overrule them? **(ethical knowledge, insight/imagination)**.

The clinical reasoning process

The patient's needs for an operation have not changed but the resources available have **(propositional adaptation knowledge)**. The need for a critical care bed is essential **(propositional knowledge)**. It is the surgeon's responsibility to ensure a suitable post-operative bed is available for his patient before the operation is started **(procedural knowledge)**. The risks of infection with MRSA to this patient include the risk of death **(propositional medical knowledge)**. As the clinical solution to this, the surgeon cancels the case, but the underlying problems remain. The patient still needs to be found a suitable bed and the risky Trust policy will, without some intervention, continue. What should the consultant now do? **(ethical knowledge, propositional and procedural knowledge)**.

The scenario of the wider issues of clinical practice *continued:*

The deliberative process

He recognizes that he has fulfilled his responsibilities to the patient in this particular context but there is an urgent need to explore and change the Trust MRSA policy **(procedural improvisation knowledge)**. His heart sinks, as he knows that this will incur more meetings, diplomacy and time **(experiential knowledge)**. He gathers his thoughts into an argument that will persuade non-surgeons to change the protocol **(evidence-based knowledge)**. This involves his knowledge of his professional responsibilities, Trust systems and policies, Trust personnel, and the current spotlight in which MRSA is being discussed in the media. He talks to the key members of staff involved and a meeting is set up to review the protocols **(procedural improvisation knowledge)**. The particular aim is to ensure that the protocol indicates that the consultant in charge of the case is informed of such problems before the patient is admitted **(professional knowledge, practice-generated knowledge, ethical knowledge, evidence-based knowledge)**.

Comment

This scenario emphasizes and demonstrates the fact that the knowledge that surgeons use is not confined merely to their clinical practice but also relates to their wider responsibilities.

End note

This chapter has looked at knowledge the surgeon draws upon in practice, and illustrated this by reference to examples from diagnosis, broad treatment areas, and wider clinical issues. These examples offer ways of both teaching and assessing such knowledge in those contexts. The following chapter focuses on the clinical thinking, and practice knowledge inherent in technical and operative procedures and in particular it looks at the assessment of them.

Chapter 10

Assessing technical and operative procedures in the context of teaching and learning surgery

Introduction

Understanding formative and summative assessment for technical and operative procedures

Preparation for technical and operative assessment: the learner's perspective

Preparation for technical and operative assessment: the teacher's perspective

The need for a structured programme for learning and teaching technical and operative procedures

Setting a bespoke programme for the learner

The principles of *seeing*, *doing* and *reflecting* on technical and operative procedures

The multi-disciplinary resources for teaching skills

Assessing operative competence in the clinical setting, taking holistic account of the learner's conduct

The philosophy

The Triggered Assessment

Preparation for an operative competence test in the clinical setting

Minimum requirements for operative competence assessment

A framework to aid reflection on surgical assessment

The requirements of the learner in a summative assessment

Developing understanding of assessment by exploring it in practice

The team reflective debriefing

The changing roles for the theatre team involved in summative assessment of operative procedures

Summary

Introduction

This chapter takes the reader further into our arguments about cultivating a thinking surgeon by emphasizing the inseparable relationship of knowing and thinking, with doing. It focuses particularly on the assessment of technical and operative procedures in clinical practice, which we believe needs to be put in place. With this in mind it seeks to:

❐ consider the elements involved in the preparation for technical and operative assessment;

❑   describe a new method for the summative assessment of operative competence which takes holistic account of the learner's conduct.

Understanding formative and summative assessment for technical and operative procedures

This section offers six elements that need to be taken into account in preparing for the assessment of technical and operative procedures. Following our usual principles we begin with the learner.

Preparation for technical and operative assessment: the learner's perspective

When young surgeons start a new clinical attachment today, the most common question asked of them by their new consultant is: Have you passed the examinations? What can you do? meaning What operations are you proficient in? How many of them have you done? This last question, whilst aimed at judging what the trainee may need to go on to learn, is mainly levelled at knowing what the trainee may be left to do straight away as a working (as distinct from a learning) member of the department. The mindset of the consultant is often on how to ensure that the work of the department is done rather than attending to teaching clinical and operative skills. The learner is left to concentrate on passing the examination but is also left thinking: 'Surely I must be allowed to do more in order to learn, to be useful, to demonstrate my skills, and to contribute to the service within my capabilities'.

In the past and throughout the life of the NHS, surgical trainees have always carried a significant responsibility for attending to the operative workload of both the emergency and elective care of patients. They were immersed in doing things in clinical practice. They were assessed in an informal way by the consultants they worked with. Until recently, they were valued members of the hospital staff. However, today's culture, aimed at maintaining the activity of the organisation, has undermined this. The ever-diminishing status of the SHO in surgery is a typical example and they now have few chances to demonstrate informally their operative ability. They may be forgiven for thinking that their supervision has been eroded to the point of serious danger.

Young surgeons are the bedrock of the surgical services of the future. They must be encouraged to engage in activities that will make them safe surgeons. They must develop a mindset which drives them to seek opportunities to demonstrate their technical and operative ability in order to justify their progression in surgery, as well as provide evidence for clinical governance. They must prepare to be able:

❑   to articulate clearly their current knowledge and achievements with evidence of clear self-knowledge;

❑   to immerse themselves thoroughly in clinical and operative practice;

❐   to create a professional relationship with their consultant colleagues;

❐   to recognize that no one can learn for them, especially on how to do an operation;

❐   to demonstrate a disciplined approach to their operative experiences, how they learn from them, and how they record that learning;

❐   to demonstrate a willingness to work as part of the extended surgical team;

❐   to talk and reflect with a range of members of the theatre team about their progress;

❐   to know what they have to learn and to what standard;

❐   to demonstrate their understanding of being a postgraduate learner, which brings with it the responsibilities:

  • of self-directed learning as distinct from being taught;

  • of problem-solving (learners need to be rehearsed in this at all stages in patient care);

  • for learning about the clinical condition *before they come to theatre*;

  • for learning about the anatomy of the procedure or the operation *before they come to theatre*;

  • for practising frequently and *before they come to theatre*, specific skills like knot tying and instrument handling;

  • for understanding modern medical educational practice and the need to maintain an educational portfolio;

  • for knowing about the traditional ways of doing things and critiquing these;

  • for recognizing the knowledge they are using, and learning to build on that knowledge;

  • for understanding the role of intuition which needs to be pinpointed, highlighted and discussed;

  • for exploring professional judgement;

  • for clarifying what expertise actually is.

Preparation for technical and operative assessment: the teacher's perspective

Consultant surgeons make tacit (and not always correct) assumptions about their trainees from the very first meeting. They review and build on these as they observe the trainee in the ward, in the outpatients and in the operating theatre. It takes time however to let them do things independently, and comments made by consultants echo the following: 'I don't have time to get to know the trainee and so I'm reluctant to let them do things'; 'I need to have at least six months with them to feel confident to let them operate unsupervised on my patients'.

Traditionally the decision to allow a trainee to operate on a patient is made by individual consultants, each making their own independent assessment, which is not recorded or used as currency by the trainee in their next job. There is no explicit agreed understanding of how consultants come to this decision. This works against the progress of the learner who may have already gained many skills in previous jobs but who will be expected to repeatedly demonstrate them to a new consultant in order to gain their confidence. The absence of a robust and reliable process of clinical and operative assessment therefore hinders the progress of the learner. The major changes to hospital practice with respect to the EWTD, consultant contracts, targets and regulation, have destabilized consultants and their approach to teaching. Consultants may be forgiven for thinking that they alone are responsible for teaching trainees and that with no officially allocated time for this they are fighting an uphill battle from which it might be better to walk away.

The surgical profession of the future depends on today's surgical teachers. It requires them not merely to recognize their responsibility in surgical education and training but actively to create a safe practicum that will achieve this (see Chapter 4). In preparing to teach technical and operative skills, surgical teachers must develop for themselves and share with trainees an understanding of:

- thinking like a surgeon;
- knowing the curriculum;
- clinical practice and the role of the multi-disciplinary team in teaching, learning and assessment;
- integrating propositional knowledge (especially anatomy and its variations) with physical sensory knowledge learned in practice;
- linking the clinical observations of diseases in patients with previously learned images of diseases in organs, in order to ensure that clinical features and underlying basic scientific knowledge are clearly integrated;
- the distinction between careful perception and unfocused observation, because using all one's sensory abilities is far more complex than merely watching;
- how to negotiate what needs to be taught during the given clinical attachment;
- the need for discipline in maintaining and using the educational portfolio;
- the need to break down operations into their component parts;
- the principles of formative and summative assessment;
- the importance of operative competence assessment which is both a formative and summative process, the latter serving as evidence to allow trainees to operate as the lead surgeon *during* training.

In respect of this last point, enabling the trainee to experience being the lead surgeon will require of the profession a valid and robust process of operative competence assessment. In the light of the demands of the Clinical Negligence Scheme for Trusts and for trainees to sign off their competencies, this has become an imperative.

The need for a structured programme for learning and teaching technical and operative procedures

The curriculum for the surgical programme will set out the stages and the range and complexity of technical procedures to be learned. This is the guide for learner and teacher to enable them to plan a specific programme for each trainee. However, surgical practice is not a static practice. New knowledge is being added each month and new technical procedures and operations are introduced into practice on a regular basis. Curriculum developers will be aware of this, but learners too need to note such changes and recognize that the syllabus must change to reflect these developments.

Examples of change in operative practice over the last twenty years include the introduction of drugs to treat peptic ulcer disease, which have eliminated the need for surgical intervention for chronic peptic ulcer disease, and laparoscopic surgery, which has transformed the operation for gallstones and threatens to become the norm for other operations such as hernia repair and appendicectomy. Surgical teachers need to take account of these changes so that they do not compromise the learner by falling into the trap illustrated by the story *The Sabre-Tooth Curriculum*. Here, revering established traditions of practice (teaching paleolithic learners how to scare away sabre-tooth tigers to defend their settlements) obscures for the educator the need to take intelligent account of changes in real practice (the extinction of the tigers not prompting the dropping of this subject within the curriculum) (see Benjamin, 1939).

A structured programme for learners in each attachment is essential so that they understand what they have to do and are able to plan accordingly. The curriculum must indicate the criteria for summative operative competence assessment and teachers and learners must be fully aware of these.

Setting a bespoke programme for the learner

Learners will each bring their own unique autobiography and curriculum vitae to the programme. Developing a bespoke programme for each one is therefore a necessity. It must aim to address the requirement of the curriculum and avoid excessive repetition at the expense of increasing the range of the learning opportunities. The good judgement of both teacher and learner will be necessary to ensure a rounded and well-balanced programme.

The principles of seeing, doing and reflecting on technical and operative procedures

Learners first need to see a procedure before doing it. However, they must develop (and therefore the teacher must model and highlight) a disciplined approach to how they observe and how they think about what they are observing and what they can learn from it. They must mentally prepare for how they will develop their capability in particular procedures and how their abilities will transpose to other aspects of their practice. Unfocused observation is unprofitable and therefore unacceptable.

Setting a short time aside following observation in order to record in writing what they have learned and to use it as a foundation for further learning is fundamental to getting the most out of such experiences. It will provide a record of what they are learning, how they are progressing and what they must go on to learn. Experienced surgeons, who have not thought about being a teacher as distinct from being a surgeon, may not see the point of this. They may not recognize that during their long years of training they developed such disciplines, which they now follow unconsciously, in their heads. The length of time they had in training allowed for this slower way of learning. The shorter time learners now have to develop the range and depth of operative skills requires them to be able to maximise every learning opportunity in ways not previously considered. Reflective writing, done intelligently and rigorously, will enhance the clinical and operative experiences.

Those aspiring to become surgeons should be encouraged to see and take part in learning the operative skills of surgery from the moment that they seriously consider a career in surgery. This will normally be during their undergraduate course or in the foundation years of postgraduate practice. They need to move quickly into the role of First Assistant and become competent in doing parts of operations. Learning a different part of the operation in an incremental way will eventually provide them with all the components to perform the whole operation. Keeping a learning account (in their educational portfolio) of their developing skills and experience would be motivating and confidence-building.

Underpinning this skilled performance, however, are propositional and procedural knowledge. With increasing confidence in operative skills the learner must build into their learning and their writing the wider aspects of the context of their practice.

In summary therefore, we can say that the following are essential.

- ❐ Learners must immerse themselves in all aspects of technical and operative practice.
- ❐ Observation of this practice must enable the learning surgeon to see, analyze and interpret all that occurs.
- ❐ Professional conversation between surgical teacher and learner during operative procedures is a vital part of the learning process with increasing emphasis on the learner's language.
- ❐ Reflective accounts of the learning and understanding must be rigorous, and surgical teachers must ensure this.
- ❐ Surgeon educators must help learners to investigate examples of professional judgment in operative practice.

The multi-disciplinary resources for teaching skills

The NHS is the biggest employer in Europe. As a source of learning opportunities for teachers and learners, its potential is enormous. The multi-disciplinary theatre team, which includes the learner surgeon, is just one microcosm of the organisation which is available to contribute to the development of the young surgeon. Nurses have always played a role in the development of doctors but now there is a much wider community who can contribute. Over the past ten years there has been a tendency to think that consultant surgeons must do all the teaching themselves, but this is neither possible nor appropriate.

Innovative consultants have always harnessed help from their colleagues in other disciplines to support teaching. Every member of the theatre team has something to offer. Offerings range from how the theatre runs, to specific skills and how various instruments and machines work.

Each member is also a model of how to conduct oneself in theatre. The Chester Multi-disciplinary Operating Theatre Study Group has been engaged like others (see Vallis, Hesketh, and MacPherson, 2004) in encouraging the development of new opportunities for learning surgeons by utilizing the whole team in their education. Currently, the theatre nursing staff rarely, if ever, has a formal role in teaching surgeons. As a result of the Chester project, local plans are being put in place to involve young surgeons in the professional activities of their nursing colleagues (Fazey, *et al*, personal communication); see also Résumé to Part one, p. 119). This should allow a better understanding and the availability of new learning opportunities. The Operating Department Practioners (ODPs) too have a great deal to offer with respect to equipment, theatre protocols, and manual handling and theatre safety (McHale, *et al*, personal communication). It is planned that a lead ODP with an understanding of the surgical curriculum will play a role in teaching young surgeons. The developing role of the Surgical Care Practitioner, who will mirror some of the areas of practice of the junior surgeons, should be seen as providing an opportunity to increase shared learning rather than as a threat, and as offering exciting new opportunities in surgical education.

In addition to supporting the surgeon's learning in theatre, we believe that the entire team also needs to be involved in the summative assessment of operative competence. The team's understanding of the purposes of the assessment must be very clear. The following section sets this out in detail.

Assessing operative competence in the clinical setting, taking holistic account of the learner's conduct

The philosophy

We have already argued that assessment must be part of the process of teaching and learning and must be carried out in real practice. We concede that no assessment process aiming to test performance in the real clinical setting, will ever be free from the effect of the opinions of assessors and those being assessed. We do not believe that summative assessment carried out in a simulator resolves this problem. After all, it would never be considered as suitable to carry out the driving test in a simulator, so why should we consider it for assessing surgeons? Assessment in clinical practice asks the learner to demonstrate their ability in the environment in which they will ultimately work. It must be rigorous and fair, with processes and reasoning being transparent to all, the process being part of routine practice and therefore cost neutral.

A surgeon educator, who knows the learner well, and who has responsibility for their development, must take the lead and have the final say in summative assessment. Whilst success in the operative skills will be an absolute requirement of such an assessment (being necessary but not sufficient to pass), the learner's conduct considered holistically must also influence the outcome. The views of other members of the team must contribute to this, and at all times during such assessment the safety of the patient must be protected. Close supervision of the learner by the consultant as well as by other supportive members of the team, is essential. Without such an assessment, a learning surgeon will never be able to tell a patient how their craft has been learned, tested and developed.

The philosophy of a rigorous summative operative competence assessment is based on the fact that it is:

- both a summative and a formative assessment of the learner;
- an holistic assessment of the learner;
- a demonstration of leadership by the consultant supervisor in managing the process;
- a demonstration of leadership in theatre by the learner before and during the assessment;
- carried out in a context-specific environment (i.e. the real clinical setting);
- safe for the patient;
- based on using multiple perspectives on the conduct of the learner given by, for example:
  - a consultant surgeon with knowledge of the learner;
  - an anaesthetist;
  - a nurse;
  - another person, for example an ODP, or another doctor;
- an opportunity for the learner to demonstrate the pinnacle of their achievement in respect of one of the required procedures for the attachment, and how their capability relates to the standard set in the curriculum;
- able to demonstrate increasing development of the learner in respect of the requirements of the curriculum;
- able to provide a clear record of evidence of competence of the learner to meet the needs of clinical governance;
- able to provide information for teacher and learner to discuss and plan future educational opportunities and career progress;
- a transparent process of assessment which is open to scrutiny by anyone who wishes to be reassured about it.

The Triggered Assessment

In 2003, the Royal College of Surgeons of England, for the first time in its history, piloted a process of operative competence assessment, which was based on the criteria described above. It evolved from the deliberations of many surgeons, other educators and college staff who were writing a curriculum for basic surgical training (The General Professional Practice of Surgery or GPPS). The above philosophy was used to guide surgeons to clarify the processes of teaching and assessment that they routinely used, and to refine these into a formalized transparent process suitable for summative assessment, which was called 'Triggered Assessment' (TA). The term was derived from the fact that the assessment was triggered by the SHO learner, once s/he could demonstrate evidence of suitable experience in a particular technical or operative skill. In presenting this evidence to their surgeon educator they triggered the need for a summative assessment to be scheduled. The outcome of such an assessment provides evidence in the portfolio for the trainee and the educator of both formative and summative development of the trainee and is the basis for planning further development. By this means a range of surgical skills with increasing complexity is experienced and evidenced by the trainee.

GPPS was piloted in two deaneries in 2003 and subjected to an educational evaluation over a six-month period (Brigley, *et al*, 2003). This was preceded by an evaluation of the standard training programme for SHOs, which provided a comparison between the old and the new. The views and ideas of consultants and surgical trainees about this new curriculum and the operative competence test in particular, was the key focus of the research. The study unearthed in the standard programme the opportunistic nature of clinical practice and its opportunities for learning surgical skills at the present time. By comparison, GPPS was seen to give direction to SHOs and their teachers of what, how, and how well (to what standard) SHOs should be progressing in order to satisfy the requirements of the programme. It was seen by SHOs in surgery and their consultants as an improvement on what currently happened (Brigley, *et al*, 2003 and Brigley, *et al*, 2004). This is because it clearly identified what SHOs need to do in order to progress and described clearly the ways they could demonstrate this. The research report inevitably recorded everyone's anxieties about the availability of the time and facilities necessary to allow this to happen. It urged the development of expert surgeon teachers to embrace and develop it. The research team and those in the study applauded the educational ideals and the idea of a summative skills test, carried out in the real context of clinical practice.

Preparation for an operative competence test in the clinical setting

All summative tests have to be prepared for by both learner and teacher. No athlete would expect to be successful without careful, well thought out and planned preparation, including observation of themselves on video in order to learn more about how to refine their techniques. We have itemized below nine key requirements for a successful skills assessment in clinical practice. Following this we describe an assessment in the operating theatre, but would stress the fact that the process is equally adaptable to the assessment of technical procedures in any clinical environment, including outpatients and the ward.

Minimum requirements for operative competence assessment

The following nine requirements are the minimum for success of this process and are: a curriculum which specifies levels of ability for assessment; a syllabus; a supportive Trust management culture; a consultant surgeon assessor who understands the detail of the process; a live clinical setting and a supportive multi-disciplinary team; the learner's log, which documents procedures learned; a learner with mature self-assessment; the full paperwork relating to TA; the importance of the learner's reflection in contributing to that assessment.

We now offer criteria related to each of these requirements.

A curriculum which specifies levels of ability for assessment

The following examples illustrate ways of expressing levels of ability of the learner, by indicating the type of supervision that they need when they perform technical and operative procedures. This has never previously been required, and ways of expressing levels of supervision (thereby indicating level of ability) continue to be developed.

Table 10:1 The levels of supervision and ability as described in the GPPS draft. (Reprinted with permission of The Royal College of Surgeons of England, © February 2003).

LEVEL 1	Theoretical knowledge of the procedure
LEVEL 2	Able to assist with the procedure
LEVEL 3	Able to do under close supervision
LEVEL 4	Able to do independently

The Royal College of Surgeons of England's GPPS draft curriculum first described these useful and simple levels of supervision to be used in a Triggered Assessment (see Table 10:1).

The descriptions of the range of levels were further developed for the intercollegiate draft curriculum in September 2003 (see Table 10:2). This increased the range and clarified the role of the teacher and learner with respect to supervision.

Table 10:2 The levels of supervision and ability. (The Royal Colleges of Surgeons' Curriculum Framework for Surgery. Reprinted with permission of The Royal College of Surgeons of England, © September 2003).

Level	Definition
1.	Teacher showing: learner assisting
2.	Learner doing: teacher assisting
3.	Learner doing: teacher watching
4.	Learner doing: teacher within theatre environs
5.	Learner doing: teacher in the hospital
6.	Learner doing: teacher at home

In Table 10:3 below, we offer our further development of this, which brings knowing and thinking into relationship with doing, so that it becomes a holistic process taking account of those issues we have discussed in Chapters 7, 8 and 9.

Table 10:3 Our adaptation of levels of supervision and ability.

Level of	KNOWING	DOING technical and operative skills	THINKING
1.	Having to ask or be told	Teacher showing: Learner assisting	Clinical reasoning
2.	Knowing where to find the knowledge but not really knowing it	Learner doing: teacher assisting	
3.	Confident in knowledge and able to demonstrate that knowledge	Learner doing: teacher watching	
4.	Able to understand and use that knowledge	Learner doing: teacher within theatre environs	Clinical reasoning and deliberation
5.	Able to develop that knowledge and build on it during practice	Learner doing: teacher in the hospital	Clinical reasoning, deliberation and practical wisdom
6.	Able to research and critique that knowledge and use it wisely	Learner doing: teacher available by phone	Excellent professional judgements

A syllabus

This indicates the range and complexity of generic and specialty technical and operative procedures (including part procedures), which need to be learned. Examples of this for surgeons are to be found in The General Professional Practice of Surgery, Draft February 2003 and The Joint Committee for Higher Surgical Training Curriculum, 2004 (http://curriculum.jchst.org/pilot/).

A supportive Trust Management culture

Crucial to a successful assessment process is a Trust culture which understands the purpose and value of the assessment with respect to patient safety. Further discussion of this can be found in Playdon, (2004).

A consultant surgeon assessor who understands the detail of the process

Consultant surgeon assessors well versed in the detail and responsibility of the summative assessment, and its place in teaching and learning, are essential. Particularly, they need to recognize that this assessment has a role to play as part of the entire educational process of the attachment. They must understand the educational and regulatory requirements of the processes and be well rehearsed in leading the assessment.

A live clinical setting and a supportive multi-disciplinary team

The assessment must take place within a routine operating list. The theatre team must understand the educational and regulatory requirements in relation to the learner, and be well rehearsed in the summative assessment. The theatre environment must be made safe for the assessment process, in particular for the patient as well as the person being assessed.

The learner's log which documents procedures practised ready for the assessment

An essential part of this process involves learners in creating a log of the procedures they have completed on the way to the summative assessment. The educational agreement between the assessor and the learner at the start of an attachment should have set a plan for this. It provides evidence of learning which should, as appropriate, include skills learned in both laboratory and clinical practice.

A learner with mature self-assessment

The learner should present to their consultant the case for triggering the assessment, either during a professional conversation or by submitting a written request. This statement allows the teacher to assess the thinking processes of the learner about their self-assessment. Any oral agreement should be carefully logged.

The full paperwork relating to triggered assessment

We have adapted the Triggered Assessment Form found in the RCS England GPPS draft curriculum. It usefully indicates the knowing, thinking and doing elements and their relationship to the process.

Table 10:4 Triggered Assessment Form for theatre.

Learner's Name:	Attachment number:	Specialty:

Surgeon/Medical Educator:	Procedure/Operation:	Date:

Within each of the following three sections, the learner must:	Surgeon/Medical assessors comments recorded during the assessment	Outcome: Satisfactory (S) or Needs Improvement (NI)
1. Preparation (for operation/intervention) Communicate appropriately with the other members of the team Greet the patient appropriately and identify the patient with the notes and take/check consent/therapy planned Confirm appropriateness of operation/treatment Confirm with patient the need to proceed Confirm/mark the operative/therapy site/side appropriately Prepare, position and drape the patient correctly Demonstrate the attitudes and professional manner appropriate for a surgeon		
2. Intervention DOING: Procedure/Operation/Intervention Perform the procedure/operation/intervention according to specialty guidelines KNOWING: Be able verbally to demonstrate appropriate propositional knowledge during the procedure THINKING: Be able to demonstrate appropriate clinical thinking during the procedure Demonstrate the attitudes and professional manner appropriate for a surgeon		
3. Post-procedure/Operation/Intervention Dress the wound/treatment site appropriately Make record and post-treatment plan Check patient in post-procedure Demonstrate the attitudes and professional manner appropriate for a surgeon		

The importance of reflection in contributing to the assessment

At the end of the assessment, the learner will be required to write a personal reflective account of the assessment. The other key assessors will also be required to do likewise. The learner will present an account to the team who will contribute their versions at the team debriefing. The final decision of the consultant will take account of this. We offer below a framework for reflecting on an operative assessment, which has five main sections, and suggested questions for each section. This is intended as an aid to reflection, and as learners become proficient in its use we would expect them to use it as a rule of thumb which provides guidance, but which does not have to be followed slavishly, providing that the level and depth of critique that it prompts is maintained.

A framework to aid reflection on surgical assessment

A: The context

- ❏ Reflections on your preparation for the triggered assessment
- ❏ What did you do to prepare for this assessment?
- ❏ How could you have improved your preparation for this assessment?
- ❏ What key professional judgements did you make at this stage?

B: Preparation for technical and operative procedures

Key elements of assessment: communication with team/patient; consent; marking and positioning patient; professionalism.

Reflections on the first section of the assessment.

- ❏ What were the key things you did?
- ❏ What were the key aspects of your clinical thinking?
- ❏ What medical/surgical knowledge did you draw on?
- ❏ What key patterns emerged (if any)?
- ❏ How might others (professionals/patients) involved in the practice see it overall?
- ❏ Comment on the oral language used between self and fellow professionals
- ❏ What key professional judgements did you make?

C: Procedure/operation/intervention

Key elements of assessment: doing; thinking; knowing; professionalism.

- ❏ What were the key things you did?
- ❏ What were the key aspects of your clinical thinking?
- ❏ What medical/surgical knowledge did you draw on?

☐ What new knowledge did you create during the event?
☐ What theories/expectations did you bring to the event? (Were they correct?)
☐ What moral and ethical issues were raised for you by this experience?
☐ What key professional judgements did you make?

D: Post-procedure/operation/intervention

Key elements of assessment: recording the event; managing post-procedure care; professionalism.

☐ What were the key things you did?
☐ What were the key aspects of your clinical thinking?
☐ What medical/surgical knowledge did you draw on?
☐ What new knowledge did you create during the event?
☐ What theories/expectations did you bring to the event? (Were they correct?)
☐ What moral and ethical issues were raised for you by this experience?
☐ What key professional judgements did you make?

E: Overview of the assessment

☐ What have you learnt from this assessment so far?
☐ How does it relate to past experiences, and how will it relate to future ones?
☐ What would you say about your professionalism?
☐ What issues and practices need further development?
☐ What theories might be developed for future action?
☐ How will your clinical thinking, medical knowledge and medical action specific to this practical procedure be modified in the light of this experience?
☐ What do you need to find out more about? How will you do this?
☐ What explorations/investigations of future practice might now be planned?
☐ What new insights about yourself have you gained from this?

The requirements of the learner in a summative assessment

The operative competence summative assessment is an opportunity for learning surgeons to demonstrate their capability. It will be a key part of their educational portfolio and provide a guide to further development as well as evidence of what they have learned to do. The following five sections describe the various parts of the assessment.

Pre-operative assessment and consent

A minimum requirement of anyone who undertakes surgery is to understand the indications and consent processes of advising a patient that they need an operation. It requires propositional and procedural knowledge as well as the ability to communicate with the patient and other people involved in the process.

Communication with the team throughout the procedure

The learning surgeon doing the operation becomes, for the duration of the assessment process, the leader of the team. The ability to manage and lead is part of what is being assessed. It is important that examinees recognize this and can act in such a capacity, demonstrating their understanding of the responsibilities that this places on them.

Carrying out the technical/operative procedure

This is the heart of the process. The standard of the technical and operative performance will usually be set by the surgical specialty for the procedure being tested. Learner and consultant must know what these are and take account of their requirements. They must also agree before the start that they are both clear about the level of supervision to be aimed for and whether it is for the whole or part of the operation. On the day, any variation in the procedure, due to unusual anatomy or more extensive disease than anticipated, must be taken account of by the assessing consultant in their final deliberations.

Arranging post-operative care

Doing the operation requires the surgeon to plan appropriate post-operative care. This will be taken account of by the assessor as will recording the details of the operation and writing letters to other colleagues needing to know about the case.

Participating in the team reflective debrief

The multiple perspectives are essential to avoid the consultant assessor's (possible) biased opinion. The aim here is fair assessment. We have already provided an example of a framework to assist this process.

The final outcome of the assessment will be made by the surgeon assessor who will take account of:

- specific comments to the teacher by key team members e.g. the senior nurse, ODP or an anaesthetist, on the performance of the learner as well as comments from the learner themselves;
- their own personal observation;
- self-assessment of the learner as evidenced in their reflective account.

The assessor is responsible for ensuring that the record of the assessment process is kept, as well as ensuring the next step in the learner's programme is planned.

Developing understanding of assessment by exploring it in practice

We have been running a project at the Countess of Chester NHS Foundation Trust to explore with the whole theatre team the feasibility of the TA. It has been supported by a grant from the Ursula Keys Charity. The project has involved two operating theatre teams coming together to learn about SHOs in surgical training, and in particular the assessment of their operative competence. We have used the GPPS draft curriculum as our curriculum model. Joining the project was entirely voluntary, but was embraced with great enthusiasm and commitment by doctors, nurses and ODPs. The process involved seminars, clinical observations including video-recording, and reflective writing and discussion. It has uncovered more knowledge about the working of clinical teams than the intended aims of the project.

The key things that we have learned are that the TA is feasible. It requires a committed and well informed team led by a capable consultant. As in any educational process, we have learned more than we expected and our findings will inevitably lead to further refinement of our clinical activities, not only those related to the assessment. One significant development is the recognition of what the theatre team can offer as teachers of surgeons in training, and we plan to take these ideas further. The team reflective debriefing is worth reporting and is described further below. One of the unexpected findings was the significant need for the change of roles by the various members of the team as they took part in the assessment (as opposed to when they were teaching the SHO). We discuss this below, under each member of the team.

The team reflective debriefing

The team reflective debriefing was at first daunting for the SHOs. They bravely took on the challenge. They wrote down their account of their assessment immediately following the operation, using Strands as a guide to their reflective writing (see Fish and Twinn, 1997; and also Chapter 5, p. 71). They met with the theatre team later and led the discussion by presenting their account of events and their feelings about them. The whole team contributed their reflective account and comparisons between accounts revealed widely different foci of attention by different members of the team. It provided a rich account of events, much of which would have been missed if the dialogue had been between the consultant and the SHO only.

The SHOs soon discovered that in a supportive atmosphere (involving both critique as well as accolade) they found a voice to explain how they felt and how sometimes they did not seem to be getting through to consultants! Comparisons of reflective writing on the same event clearly demonstrated a quite different mindset and area of thinking between consultant and SHO. For example, Linda de Cossart's accounts were often about managing what was happening outside the operating theatre whilst the SHO gave careful descriptions of the techniques and their ability to handle tissues. The team were able to break down barriers and encourage wider deliberation. The videos emphasized the focus of concentration of the SHO on the operative procedure almost to the exclusion of events unfolding around them. This was particularly so the more inexperienced they were, and the findings gave insight into the need for sensitivity to the level of experience of the learner in such assessments. A wider range of their focus of attention would be expected as they became more experienced. We were all left in no doubt that this team environment was essential to the process and added to the quality of the assessment of the SHO. Care of patients in the operating theatre can only be improved by such measures.

The changing roles for the theatre team involved in summative assessment of operative procedures

The discovery that each individual team member's role changed during the formal assessment as compared to when they were supporting the SHO's learning, surprised us. On reflection the need for such changes should have been obvious and underpins the need for there to be a committed team approach to this type of assessment. We describe below the effect on various members of the team.

From supervising consultant to examiner

The surgeon educator is responsible for setting up the assessment. This must ensure that the environment is safe for both patient and trainee. They are responsible for preparing appropriate members of the theatre team to take an active part in the assessment as well as the reflective debriefing. The patient too should be taken into the planning and be reassured that this is *not* an experiment but part of a well tried pattern of surgical development which has been going on since teaching surgery began. The only difference is (and this ought to be reassuring) that the assessor, the learner and the whole theatre team are all prepared as never before for this formal process of assessment.

Having prepared the scene, the consultant assessor, at the time of the assessment must:

- not engage in a teaching role during this procedure;
- not be scrubbed but must maintain a passive supervisory role (being ready to help should there be a need);
- only ask questions that enlighten them to the thinking and the knowledge being used by the trainee;
- not engage in distracting conversation;
- have appropriate paperwork suitably organized;
- not let the paperwork distract them.

From learner to leader

The assessment team is observing the trainee as leader of the theatre team as well as a technically skilled operator. During the piloting of TAs we were surprised that the trainees needed to be prompted to act in the role of leader. Their natural tendency was to continue in the role of learner, probably because the consultant was in the operating room. Some learners found this quite a revelation and it was a significant, emancipating experience for them once they had recognized it. It is essential that in preparing for the assessment, trainees recognize their changing role and practise it.

Learners therefore need to:

❏ understand the process and prepare for the assessment;
❏ ensure that their communications with their supervisor are clear and accurate and that the case booked is appropriate;
❏ recognize their role on the day and take the lead, acting within the bounds of their profession;
❏ recognize the importance of communication with the rest of the team, both in preparation for the assessment and during the assessment;
❏ understand how the team can support them;
❏ be able to do the operation;
❏ be able to demonstrate their theoretical knowledge of the clinical case;
❏ be able to explain their clinical thinking related to this and other similar cases.

From experienced first assistant to obedient helper

An assistant must be available for the operation and this must not be the consultant assessor. This fact emerged during the first TA, when the consultant turned up, not expecting to assist, while everyone else expected them to. A first assistant was quickly found, but then discovered that the role was not the same as when they were assisting during a normal learning process. The orientation of the first assistant has to change during a TA. It is important to look to the lead surgeon (who is being assessed) and respond to their instructions rather than being pro-active and moving into the lead whenever the learner seems to hesitate. The assistant must of course use their experience to ensure the safety and fairness of the process, but they must give the floor to the SHO being assessed. The level of experience of first assistants will obviously vary in different circumstances, but there will be occasions when the assistant will be more senior than the lead (for example if an SHO is being assisted by a registrar or even another consultant). The assistant must not stand back and ignore a situation when it seems that the learner is having difficulty but they will need to recognize the difference between difficulty which is being managed safely and difficulty where the learner is in trouble. This will require the assistant to avoid teaching and become an obedient helper who exercises common sense. We have found that once this has been understood, most who take the first assistant's role have no further problems.

The assistant must:

❏ understand the process and be prepared for their role in it;
❏ learn to be the passive and obedient helper;
❏ adjust their actions according to the complexity of the procedure;
❏ learn for themselves about their own understanding of the process with respect to their professional development.

From pro-active scrub assistant to reactive/responsive scrub assistant

The scrub assistant is normally very pro-active in their routine involvement in an operation and during the SHOs learning. But during an assessment they must support the learner. They must not however run the case. The learner must be allowed to demonstrate their ability to guide the scrub assistant in how they wish the case to proceed. This of course will be the situation later in real life when the experienced learner is required to work with a scrub assistant whom they have not previously met and who is unfamiliar with the case. The scrub assistant ideally should be one of the designated theatre team members who understands the process and who will take part in the reflective debriefing. The consultant surgeon assessor will take heed of their comments on the conduct of the surgeon being assessed.

The scrub practitioner must therefore:

- be fully briefed and acquainted with the process by attending an educational programme for this purpose;
- have previously attended a TA as an observer;
- be prepared to support the learner;
- be able to take part in the reflective debriefing;
- be able to provide fair comment, supported by their observations on the case to the consultant assessor;
- command respect from the rest of the theatre team.

From frenetic theatre team to supporting calm environment

Operating theatres are noisy and full of activity even during operations. Modern surgeons tend to listen to music during a surgical procedure and often engage in conversation unrelated to the operation being performed. For the purposes of the assessment the theatre environment must be as calm as possible as there will be no getting away from the fact that the learner will be nervous. Undue interruption and talk must be avoided. This will usually require the most senior member of the theatre team to ensure this. It may well require notices to prevent entry to the theatre by others not involved in the assessment. These arrangements will provide a consistent theatre environment for all assessments.

The operating theatre (or any other clinical environment for that matter) when it is in the context of an assessment must provide:

- a safe environment for patient and the surgeon being assessed;
- a team that knows the requirements of the assessment;
- a team with experience, respect for and commitment to the process.

From clinical anaesthetist to supporter and observer of the learner surgeon

The anaesthetist is present in the operating theatre for all operations performed under general anaesthetic and for some complex procedures performed under regional and local anaesthetic. They have the opportunity to observe surgeons and make comparisons between a range of different surgeons. They are from a different discipline of medicine. They too, however, need to understand the curriculum and the requirements of the assessment and the multi-disciplinary environment in which it happens. As medical practitioners from a different specialty from surgeons, anaesthetists are an important resource for this assessment.

To prepare for such a role anaesthetists would have a responsibility to:

- understand the curriculum;
- be versed in the assessment process;
- be committed to playing a full role in the assessment;
- be committed to ensuring a safe and fair environment for the assessment;
- be able to take part in a reflective debriefing.

Summary

The Triggered Assessment brings into the surgical arena for the first time a strong educational enterprise of both summative and formative learning and assessment. It offers a relevant summative assessment for technical and operative competence. It attends to the creation of team spirit across various disciplines. It encourages a consistency of approach to the process and a means of harnessing the whole team in the venture. This assessment process has the versatility to be taken into other clinical settings such as the ward, the outpatients and critical care area. It has created a level of enthusiasm, motivation and new ideas amongst the team which could not have been envisaged before the project.

Chapter 11

Developing and enriching surgical teaching and learning through practitioner research

Introduction

Practitioner research: some starting points
Why should we look more deeply at our practice?
What might be involved?

Practitioner research: an overview
From scientific to educational research
The significance of practitioner research for surgeons in the 21st Century
Teacher as researcher
Developing a small-scale investigation: some general principles

Practitioner research: two useful approaches
Conversation Analysis
Case study: or 'You are a real case!'
Some helpful texts

Final end note

Introduction

We have tried to show in Part one that successful teaching and learning in the clinical setting opens up discussions about professional and educational values, involves the teacher in nurturing the learner and adopting practical and emancipatory approaches to teaching, and depends on learners making appropriate meaning out of their learning opportunities. We also pointed out that good teaching utilizes professional conversations to engage the learner in all aspects of education, and that reflective talking and writing can unpack the tacit and invisible in both the teacher's and the learner's practice. The role of assessment, we argued, is first and foremost a means of recognizing and providing lasting evidence of the learner's achievements, the pattern of which evidence can then be reviewed as a means of identifying progress (or its absence).

In Part two, we have attempted a careful analysis of both clinical thinking, and the knowledge that surgeons use, in order to illustrate how these can impact upon surgeons' clinical activities.

We have illustrated how surgical and technical procedures may be assessed. During all chapters we have drawn upon the educational understanding and principles developed in Part one to offer a range of suggestions about how teachers and learners can use these ideas, and how assessment can support them in so doing.

Teachers and learners who embark on serious educational practice will quickly be drawn to try to understand and continue to develop it. They will want to conduct evaluations of the educational value of the attachment and the broader programme, in order to continue to refine it. Such evaluation is a form of small-scale educational research. Given the central role of the professional conversation and the learner's talk in the activities discussed in almost every chapter, they will want to explore further, perhaps via Conversation Analysis, their own achievements in respect of prioritizing the learner's meaning-making. They will also want to continue to explore their practice in writing, and to develop the ideas emerging from their reflections into a larger enquiry which becomes a properly rigorous study of themselves as surgical teachers and learners or as surgeons, perhaps via Case Study Research or Action Research (which, for our purposes, are very similar in practice).

All these enterprises will also enable them not only to fulfil the need for accountability in both surgical and educational practice, but also to demonstrate that they have done so through the written evidence they collect. It is the term 'accountability', which helps us to distinguish scientific from educational research. It reminds us that we have to give an account of ourselves. The term 'account' can be associated with numbers (as in a bank account, and scientific research or investigation), or words (as in a story or narrative account of our exploits); both serve a purpose. Numbers make more sense where large-scale investigations are engaged in. Words allow us to get at the rich texture of small-scale interactions, ideas and activities. It is therefore *narratives of their practice* that practitioner researchers develop. This is not the soft option; it is in fact harder (but ultimately more enjoyable and more informative about the minutiae of practice) than any 'number-crunching' could ever be.

Setting up professionally worthwhile investigations, pursuing them rigorously and by appropriate means, and writing them up in detail, will be an important start, but only by sharing these accounts with the wider world, will this work become proper practitioner research. However, accounts of small-scale research can be relatively brief, and in the wider world can begin with ideas shared and critiqued in a learning group. This could even become a new form of Journal Club!

This final chapter opens up for the first time, some aspects of practitioner research (on which, as we said in the Introduction, our own approach to the evolution of this book has been based), and seeks to equip surgical teachers and learners to begin to explore further for themselves the educational principles, ideas, and activities that we have discussed, and to shape the development of these within their own individual practice. We also indicate at the end of the chapter further literature through which this topic can be explored, since practitioner research is a major subject within education for the professions, and one which surgeon educators and learners will increasingly need to access.

Practitioner research: some starting points

Practitioner research is usually focused on small examples of short events within professional practice and can be carried out more or less as a part of practice itself (just as education can occur as part of service). It is conducted by professionals who seek to understand and develop their own practice by exploring its finer detail.

This section seeks to whet the appetites of readers, by showing why they should engage in practitioner research (which is a particular form of educational research), and by listing the kinds of investigations that will be fruitful for them in the context of cultivating a thinking surgeon. The following section seeks to offer a more formal overview of this kind of research, in order to provide a proper understanding of the enterprise. The final section offers in detail two methods that are particularly apt for exploring the issues listed, and provides useful references for those who wish to pursue these ideas further.

Why should we look more deeply at our practice?

The surface of real practice (surgical and educational), alters its patterns as fast, as unpredictably and as uncontrollably as a jolted kaleidoscope. Retrospectively, we can never quite convey to anyone else how we saw that pattern at the time in all its texture and colour. This makes it hard to discuss and explore the fine detail, and yet it is the fine detail that is often the most significant in the development of our understanding and thus our practice. Indeed, it is virtually universally the case that what we think we see and hear in the ongoing rush of practice, is often quite misleading.

We need to slow down the processes of both surgical and educational practice, by capturing some moments in it, in ways that allow us to share and go over them a number of times, challenging what we have taken for granted and seeing our practice anew. We need to explore them (analyze and interpret them) outside the hassle and white noise of the practice setting. When we do so, we are invariably surprised at the richness of educational opportunities and understanding they open up to us. We also become more aware that we see the world through our own values and culture and that this determines the meanings we make of a situation and explains why they are not always as fully shared as we assume.

Further, professional practice, as we have seen, is complex, uncertain, morally based (because we work for vulnerable patients whose moral good we must honour), and depends upon professional judgement. How such professional judgements are made is not well understood - even by those who do it. We need to understand them better in order to refine them (for our patients' better good) and in order to defend our work in the public arena. We are the only people who can do this in respect of our own practice.

It should be noted that the intention in all this is not to prove a point, nor to collect evidence to show that we were right or wrong, but rather to uncover the problematics of professional practice in both surgery and education, and thus learn to live with and work round them, and be able to articulate why this is necessary. This becomes a fascinating study, which will turn surgical teaching and learning into an endlessly beckoning journey.

What might be involved?

The 'capturing' referred to above can be carried out in recorded form at the time (using audio tape, video or digital camera, or by the written notes of a non-participant observer), and/or by careful vivid description captured during or after the event by a participant in it. All these forms are actually subjective, of course, and are best supported by accounts or pictures from other angles. Such subjectivity is at least open (which is not the case in scientific research which claims to be objective but never can be). We offer the more formal details of how to go about this kind of practitioner research in the following section, but first we need to indicate the focus and purpose of such investigative work, and who might engage in it.

We would argue for example that surgical teachers will want to:

- ❏   interrogate examples of their own surgical practice and unearth their tacit knowledge and thinking, including professional judgement, in order to be ready to share and discuss it with learners;
- ❏   develop an evaluation of the educational value: of their own offering to the learner during the attachment (interrogate examples of their educational practice); of the attachment as a whole; and of the programme the learner is on;
- ❏   engage in reflective analysis of a particular part of a patient case in order to talk with the learner about it and also to experience what learners have to do when reflecting on a case of their own;
- ❏   capture (by audiotape/video camera) a professional conversation which reflects upon a clinical experience, and then identify a crucial few minutes of it, and analyze carefully their own spoken language, to see how well it facilitates learners as they make their own meaning of what is offered;
- ❏   consider carefully the interaction in a captured piece of professional conversation in terms of the power relationships it establishes and the space it gives the learner to be an active partner (see page 54);
- ❏   capture, listen carefully to, and explore, the learners' spoken language during their reflections on a case, in order to check on their level of understanding as it is, rather than as it seemed at the time;
- ❏   experiment with how best to set up and respond to written reflection from the learner.

And learning surgeons will want to:

- ❏   narrate, analyze and interpret various critical incidents that have an educational dimension for them, and use these to explore their own values, thinking, and knowledge as it underlies and is expressed in their actions;

- ❏ narrate, analyze and interpret a whole case study which focuses not on the patient medically but themselves educationally, and particularly on the knowledge and the thinking that drove their actions, decisions and professional judgements;
- ❏ compare their narrative with the consultant's and the patient's if possible;
- ❏ reflect on a negotiation they have needed to make with a teacher about, for example, the induction interview, negotiating study leave, and the RITA review;
- ❏ reflect on a meeting they themselves have had with a patient where consent is taken, or where some crucial information is asked for or a technical procedure has to be performed;
- ❏ explore how work actually gets done rather than how it should be done in a ward or clinic or theatre (identify the realities of practice in the practice setting and their surgical and educational implications);
- ❏ consider critically a piece of reflective writing they have done and use it as the starting point for a small-scale investigation that will illuminate a key issue that has emerged;
- ❏ contribute their own learner's perspective to the educational evaluation of the attachment and the programme they are on, by means of personal narratives.

We advocate practitioner research then (which takes a broadly 'action research' mode), for the purposes of: improving the educational evaluation of a post; exploring interaction between surgical teachers and learners; and engaging in a detailed investigation of what can be learnt from an individual patient case or a piece of reflective writing. We offer two carefully chosen research techniques, in order to provide clear and workable details of how to proceed. These are Conversation Analysis (CA), and small-scale case study research, but we set them first in the wider context of educational research generally - which context should provide the principles for designing a thorough educational evaluation.

Practitioner research: an overview

From scientific to educational research

In traditional programmes of surgical training, the research that learners carry out and that which they critique, is focused entirely upon the exploration of disease processes, their aetiology and treatment, and more interestingly, their eradication. This research is scientific in nature and falls into the positivistic research paradigm. It is based on the development of a hypothesis that is explored with the intention of proving it and so generating new propositional knowledge (theory), which others (practitioners) may choose to apply in their own work. The processes of proof and truth in science apply here. As Pring points out:

'The goal of research is normally that of producing new knowledge. There will of course, be many different motives for producing such knowledge. But what makes it research is the systematic search for conclusions about 'what is the case' on the basis of relevant evidence. Such conclusions might indeed be that of getting ever 'nearer the truth'. Hence it makes sense to see the outcomes of research to be a series of propositions that are held to be true.'

(Pring, 2000, p. 130)

The evidence for success in surgical research is based on the changes made to patient care. Highly successful research is seen as that which will affect the largest number of people. A change in the development of the researcher is almost certainly no more than a side effect. For the learner, the experience of a positive outcome will result in motivation and encouragement, but where there is a negative outcome - even where rigorous methods have been used - the result will be disappointment, and a feeling of failure and demotivation. Indeed, there is currently discussion as to whether there is value in including research in surgical training at all.

Another research approach that is more easily available for young surgeons to carry out is audit. This is designed to identify changes that need to be made to everyone's practice in a given context, and to see how to introduce such changes successfully. In both of these research approaches, the kinds of change aimed at are changes to medical practice in a very focused area. There are thus two kinds of scientific research: the experiment and the survey.

By contrast to these, educational research (which uses humanistic enquiry methods rather than scientific enquiry approaches), and which previously has had little status in surgical education, sets out to increase the researcher's understanding of his/her own educational and professional practice, and thus improve it. The development of the research is thus central. In that sense it is research carried out by the practitioner into his or her own practice (or as in the case of surgeons, into their *practices*, since the surgeon educator practises both surgery and education).

Educational research will therefore be of use to both teachers and learners. Pring notes here, that practitioner research focuses on the particular, which can also 'illuminate or be suggestive of practice elsewhere' and that:

'The conclusion [of practitioner research] is not a set of propositions but a practice or set of transactions or activities that are not true or false, but are better or worse.'

(Pring, 2000, p. 131)

Indeed, since professional knowledge (in medicine and education) has constantly to be tested out, reflected upon, and adapted to new situations, practitioner research must be examined critically and opened up to criticism and therefore needs to be made public in seminars and through publications.

There are several kinds of educational research: illuminative research, which is a small-scale version of survey research; practitioner research which includes case study; and action research which uses amongst other methods, Conversation Analysis.

The following table, which is adapted from Fish and Coles, (1998), p. 23, and Fish, (1998), p. 128-29, offers an overview of the different research traditions.

Table 11:1 The scientific and humanistic research traditions.

	Scientific research (positivistic)	Survey research (scientific/ positivistic)	Illuminative research (humanistic)	Practitioner research (humanistic)
Examples	Randomized controlled trials; experimentation	Large-scale questionnaire Audit	Complex and large-scale humanistic enquiry	Reflective and critical case study Action research
Focus	Physical world	Social world	Social world	Social world of individual practitioner (fine scale)
Main purpose	To identify truth and/or laws, so that they can be applied to practice by others	To identify hard (numerical) facts and evidence about practice on a medium to large scale in order to improve it	To identify opinion, and humanistic evidence about practice on medium to large scale in order to improve it	To understand the practice of an individual better in order to improve it
Size of world investigated	Large scale	Large to medium scale	Medium to small scale	Small scale
Key methods	Scientific Experimental Claims to be objective Uses analysis	Heavily structured questionnaire and interview Seeks to be seen as objective Uses analysis	Semi-structured interviews and non-participant observation Seeks several perspectives to gain rich 3-dimensional view Uses analysis and interpretation	Self-study via participant observation and recording, together with reflection, analysis interpretation, and appreciation, plus consideration of the understandings of others
Immediate end product	Seeks to code and measure and 'cashes out' into numbers in order to prove a point	Produces graphs and statistics to prove a point	Produces a report using words and numbers	Produces case narrative, which can be refined and extended, in which numbers may be useful evidence
Main result	New knowledge produced by researchers but applied to practice by practitioners	New knowledge produced by researchers but applied to practice by practitioners	New knowledge produced by researchers or practitioners involved and contributing to the improvement of practice	A change in understanding of the individual practitioner and a consequent refinement of that practitioner's practice
Legitimated as research by	Scientific rigour and public scrutiny via articles, or artifacts	Mathematical rigour and scrutiny via contribution to literature	Rigour of the humanistic processes and public scrutiny via contribution to literature	Rigour of case study methods, multiple perspectives and sharing of research and new practice in seminars and articles

The significance of practitioner research for surgeons in the 21st Century

In the past, when consultants argued to spend much time with trainees before they let them operate or see their special patients, they were (tacitly) concerned about getting those learners on the same wave length as themselves. The sort of educational research we are recommending in this chapter will help teacher and learner to explore where, how and why understanding is or is not being established between them, and will enable them to build more quickly this educational relationship, and establish the appropriate nurturing environment. It is all too easy for the teacher to assume that because they have spoken, the learner has learnt. Teachers who examine even very brief extracts from a recording of their dialogue with learners are often shocked by what they find.

Teacher as researcher

Professional development, practitioner research and reflective practice all converge when a member of a profession seeks to understand his/her practice better. This is the mark of an extended professional (see a comparison between an extended and restricted professional on pp. 21-22).

'The outstanding characteristics of an extended professional is [sic] a capacity for autonomous professional self-development through systematic self-study, through the study of the work of other teachers and through testing the ideas by ... research procedures [developed for use in the teaching setting].'

(Stenhouse, 1975, p. 144)

Teachers researching their practice, Stenhouse says, are concerned with understanding their own educational practice better, and seek the development of a sensitive and self-critical perspective, but do not have an aspiration towards unattainable objectivity. He adds 'illusion, assumption and habit must be continually tested. Illusion will be destroyed when disclosed. Assumptions and habits will be changed. ... The problem is one of awareness' (Stenhouse, 1975, pp. 157-8). We believe that for surgical education his words are still apt: 'A research tradition which is accessible to [surgical] teachers and which feeds teaching must be created if education is to be significantly improved' (see Stenhouse, 1975, p.165).

Developing a small-scale investigation: some general principles

This section offers some general principles that traditionally inform the design and conduct of all practitioner research. They are drawn from workshop materials that Della Fish has used successfully with health care practitioners since 1989. This will offer surgeon educators who wish to conduct robust and rigorous evaluations of the educational value of the post for their learners, a skeleton on which to build their individual investigations.

The nature of the enterprise

Understanding the nature of practitioner research is an important basis for designing the activities involved. The following can be said about it.

- ❐ The work is personal and professional rather than simply academic and abstract, and is active rather than theoretical.
- ❐ It should start with a personal question, which is focused on your practice. This should be refined so as to be able to yield to small-scale investigation which can be conducted mainly by yourself but should take account of the views, accounts, and opinions of others.
- ❐ It is a personal investigation of practice and of its underlying (tacit) personal and formal (public) theory. This is carried out by means of:
  - practical investigation using appropriate methods and tools;
  - investigating the *theory* implicit in the practice (that is theorizing one's practice);
  - wider investigation and discussion of the issues as appropriate (including reference to formal theory);
  - developing personal and informed critical reflection on the emerging issues, ideas, actions that have been created or discovered;
  - analyzing, interpreting, and appreciating what emerges;
  - being tentative rather than dogmatic;
  - seeking new understanding rather than evidence to support what is already known and, importantly;
  - striving for better educational goals/ends/ and intentions, rather than merely changing technicalities.

Exploring what this means

The word 'informed' above means taking account of the full range of perspectives on the issues at hand, including perspectives from formal theory, and the critique of one's fellows. The key methods available to a practitioner researcher (for surgeons for the purpose of beginning on practitioner research) are case study research (the study of an individual case for the educational purpose of understanding it and ourselves better), or action research (a means of investigating our practice to see whether it is as we feel it should be, and with a view to changing our practice and that of those around us). These two approaches are coming closer together but it would still be fair to say that action research seeks emancipation from current ways of seeing and working, where case study research has the slightly more modest intention of seeking to illuminate current understanding which will later lead to a change of practice. The tools include all the known investigative approaches appropriate to a small-scale enquiry that research texts offer or that common sense can devise (including discourse analysis or Conversation Analysis). Helpful texts in all these areas are listed at the end of this chapter.

The terms 'analyzing', 'interpreting' and 'appreciating' are used above in relation to the main focus of practitioner research - an event or activity (or the captured versions of these). They are being used here to mean the following.

Analysis is a process in which the components of an activity (or a process or event or its representation on paper or media) are separated into their component parts and categorized for consideration. Analysis may claim to be objective and neutral but it rests on value judgements that have to be made in order to categorize in the first place, and on assumptions including the key idea that the whole is always a simple sum of the parts. An interesting question to ask about analysis is: how far does it allow one to respond, (or prevent one from responding), holistically, to the whole activity, process or event - or to the captured record of it? Clearly, although it is open to critique, analysis must play its part in understanding an activity or event at the level of detail.

Interpretation, by contrast, treats the activity holistically. It is a process that offers a view or views of the overall nature and meaning of an activity. It is admittedly subjective, and takes account of its subjectivity in presenting its view(s). Rather than breaking the activity down into component parts, it views it overall in order to see it better, to explain it, or to try to say something about what it might mean, or what can be said about it.

By contrast to both analysis and interpretation, *critical appreciation* starts with trying to recognize and understand what the activity might mean. It is a term borrowed from the Arts. Essentially, art results from the artist seeing anew and then sharing his or her version of that vision. Critical appreciation is a process in which the artist's vision (both that which the artist was conscious of, and that which the critic sees even when the artist may not have been overtly aware of it) is recognized holistically and responded to in ways which show it has been understood. Appreciation is justified by detailed reference to the piece of art (or activity itself), and to its history and the tradition within which, or in opposition to which, it was fashioned. This process seeks to consider the activity from many points of view, seeking to set it in a context that helps to make sense of it, seeing in it meanings beyond the surface and seeing it as representative of something beyond itself. A critical appreciation, presented as a commentary, seeks to convey a sense of the achievement of the activity, set within the context of time and place and informed by some knowledge about the people involved. (The setting and the traditions within which that activity or event has occurred are significant in helping us to understand it). In addition to all that, the personal qualities, knowledge and understanding, history and traditions, values and beliefs of the critic (or appreciator) are also important, inevitably come through, and need to be acknowledged.

It will be apparent from this that the role of judge, in terms of the merit of a piece of art, comes behind the task of recognition and response. Indeed, the terms 'critic' and 'critiquing' in the context of either art or professional practice, should not connote a negative mindset, which is why we like the term 'appreciating' a professional activity or event.

Some issues about ethics

Practitioner research involves a number of professional people and sometimes vulnerable patients. This brings with it complex issues about the rights and responsibilities of all involved. This is both about the investigator's accountability, and the activities of gathering and generating evidence, storing that evidence, interpreting that evidence, and presenting the conclusions to various audiences. Since the inquiry involved is about educational matters, and will deal with problematic issues in which values are involved, it is bound to raise some issues that are controversial. What is needed therefore, is a set of ethical guidelines to work to, that ensure that everyone is treated with proper sensitivity and has their rights safeguarded.

However, we would stress that this is educational, not medical, research. It is practice development, not scientific or blue skies research. Its end is the development of educational understanding, which can only benefit patients in the longer term. We have always found that patients have been very supportive of practitioners seeking to improve practice (as for example in the work Della Fish does as an educational advisor to consultants, in the clinical setting, in Kent, Surrey and Sussex Deanery). We believe therefore that, providing the investigation follows the guidelines of the British Educational Research Association (BERA), it should be regarded as ethically sound. The BERA website address is http://www.bera.ac.uk).

Developing an investigative framework, or 'small is beautiful'

The rigour of practitioner research depends upon the robustness of the design of the investigation. Framing clearly and precisely the focus for the investigation and being able to state clearly the reasons for carrying it out are important starting points. It should be noted that this is not the same as stating and therefore constraining from the beginning, the expected end results. The following questions are offered to aid this process.

- ❐ What specifically do you want to understand better?
- ❐ What practical investigations will achieve this, given the need to carry them out in the practice setting as part of practice?
- ❐ How can several viewpoints on this focus be collected?
- ❐ What other methods and strategies can reasonably be used or created?
- ❐ What preparation is necessary before the inquiry begins (see ethics section above).

Some questions about evidence

Where positivistic research seeks data, humanistic inquiry seeks evidence. The following questions may be of use in determining how to seek, record and use the evidence in practitioner research.

- ❐ What evidence is necessary for the proper investigation of my question?
- ❐ What actually counts as evidence in this situation?
- ❐ To what end am I collecting, recording or creating this evidence?
- ❐ How can it be obtained?
- ❐ What can I properly expect access to in collecting it?
- ❐ What public and private interests are involved?
- ❐ Who has the right to know about my interpretations and conclusions?
- ❐ What is the point of collecting/creating this evidence? (Am I genuinely seeking to learn as I go, or am I looking for proof of something I already know? Am I simply after

impressing someone with figures and or the sheer weight of evidence, or am I seeking better understanding of my own practice?).

❏   Am I being open-minded about what the evidence might be telling me?

❏   Are my conclusions clear, have I opened them to challenge? Might there be another equally persuasive interpretation? Have I shared all this in an open forum?

In the light of these general principles for practitioner research, we now offer briefly two methods which we believe are of particular use to surgeon educators and their partners in learning.

Practitioner research: two useful approaches

In choosing how to investigate our practice, in order to understand it better, we need to take account of the characteristics of professional work, the nature of professional practice, and the nature of enquiry. We recommend:

❏   Conversation Analysis for the consultant brave enough to wonder whether the learning surgeon fully understands a particular professional conversation;

❏   small-scale case study starting with a critical incident, or emerging from a piece of reflective writing.

Conversation Analysis

Conversation Analysis (CA) has been developed because talk is so central to the way we conduct our lives that it has become an important focus of study in a number of disciplines. The intention of our recommended use of CA is to capture and to explore critically the language of a professional conversation, which has taken place within the clinical environs, between a learner and a teacher. There will be no patient present and any patient referred to in the conversation should not be identifiable. Only the teacher and learner therefore need to agree to the activity. The context of this conversation should be some specific learning opportunity which occurred within a clinical setting and which you are both now seeking to reflect upon. The conversation might be up to thirty minutes in length, and would be captured by audio tape, or video camera, or with the help of a fellow practitioner who acts as observer and seeks to write down as much as possible of the conversation (and whose agreement to confidentiality must be obtained).

Firstly, - before looking at the evidence you have captured - you both need, separately, to jot down your subjective view of what has been achieved in the interaction by both learner and teacher, using Chapters 3 and 4 above to remind you of key educational principles you would hope to find in it.

Secondly, you should listen to or read the whole of the recorded conversation, and seek to characterize the interaction it demonstrates, discussing this in relation to the assumptions you made about it before you looked at the evidence.

Finally, you need to choose a fruitful part of it (less than ten minutes) to focus on in detail. This may be transcribed. Any book on CA or the internet will provide the details of how to do this in a professional way (there is no one universally agreed set of conventions for this). You should do this transcription yourself, rather than ask a secretary, so as not to import further subjectivity. You should then attend to the language of the conversation in terms of the quality of the educational engagement it evidences.

The following questions may help with this.

A: Ask:

- ❏   about the teacher's and learner's intentions;
- ❏   what expectations did teacher have of learner?
- ❏   to what extent is language necessary/helpful to thinking about the task?
- ❏   how did the language lend itself to the extension of the learner's thinking about the problem?
- ❏   whose agenda did you work to?

B: Find examples of:

- ❏   learner using tentative talk and informal language to grapple with an idea;
- ❏   learner setting the agenda and/or reshaping it;
- ❏   learner being pro-active;
- ❏   learner challenging teacher;
- ❏   learner responding to teacher;
- ❏   teacher responding to and extending learner's idea(s);
- ❏   teacher supporting learner's tentative talk;
- ❏   teacher removing initiative from learner;
- ❏   teacher altering direction of discussion;
- ❏   teacher playing 'guess-what-I-am-thinking';
- ❏   real collaboration;
- ❏   real partnership in learning.

C: Identify a moment or moments when the frontiers of thinking / learning / language were being pushed forward.

You may wish to talk or write about what you have each learnt as a result of this process. We do advise the use of written transcript of the small extract that is chosen, as experience shows that there is often far more in interaction than we can notice during one hearing. Further help with all this can be found particularly in Hutchby and Woolfit, (1988 reprinted 2004); and Ten Have, (1999). The following table shows the generally accepted conventions for key elements of a transcription glossary, together with some additional comments directed at supporting this particular use of CA. We would encourage readers to use their common sense if they meet something not covered by the following, (for example, capitals can indicate shouting, and an exclamation mark, animated speech). Numbering the transactions before the speaker at the start of the first line of the utterance enables easier discussion. As in the following:

1.   Teacher: So why do you think that the patient's reaction was ….
2.   Learner: Well, I didn't expect her to …

(It will be noted in this example that the learner's agenda here is already beginning to diverge from the teacher's!).

Table 11:2 Some accepted conventions for key elements of CA.

(2.0)	The number of seconds pause or gap between or within utterances. (Where teacher is trying to encourage the learner to explore ideas through talk, the length of time teacher leaves (or does not leave) for learner to come in, is significant. Pauses in the learner's contribution might indicate a reflective learner who is thinking carefully, or lack of ability to complete the idea embarked upon, or some other reason. The utterances which follow this often give a clue about the reason, but of course it is also important to ask the learner about it.)
[ ]	Indicates the start and finish of overlapping talk (Talk is often less well structured than written prose. Turn-taking is important in professional conversation. This sign indicates something that needs to be explored further, for example, it can indicate failure of one speaker to let another in.
.hh	Indicates indrawn breath. (Is this followed by speech, or does the other speaker cut in next - and why?)
hh	Indicates an out-breath. (But how is this to be interpreted?)
(( ))	Put between these double brackets any important non-verbal activity like extraneous sounds. This can also be used for body language if it is a video that is being transcribed.
( )	Empty brackets indicate an unclear or inaudible passage
:	Colons indicate that the speaker has stretched the preceding sound or letter. What, then, does this signify?
?	Indicates a rising inflection whether the content is a question or not. (Why?)
*	Indicates strange or doubtful pronunciation. (Why?)
° °	Indicates a passage that is noticeably quieter than the surrounding talk. (Why?)

Consultants who have already engaged in this process during work with us, have found this exercise a particularly rewarding one, and some have become quite hooked on the process. We commend it to readers and hope they will enjoy the intellectual problem-solving that it engenders, and the sense of control over the development of their own practice that it provides.

Case study: or 'You are a real case!'

Case study in which a practitioner focuses on his or her own practice is a particularly useful approach to understanding and improving practice. The literature of other health care professions has much to tell us about the art of case study (see for example, Fish and Coles, 1998, and particularly Chapter 4 for a detailed exposition of case study).

Telling stories about a small incident in our practice is one way into practitioner research. We have already commended them as useful as part of the reflective processes we have been presenting earlier in the book. It is important, however, to recognize that adverse or critical incidents and the cases we develop round them that are discussed for medico-legal reasons, are not the same as critical incidents which are used for educational purposes. A critical incident which is useful educationally is one whose significance has been produced by the way we look at it. It might be something which startles, puzzles, is amusing, worrying or pleasing; or it might be a routine piece of practice which has suddenly come to the attention because it has developed habits that are questionable. Such incidents should be fully contextualized, described and then analyzed and interpreted.

Case study research, as Golby and Parrott argue persuasively, 'is uniquely appropriate as a form of educational research for practitioners to conduct', having the potential 'to relate theory and practice' and 'advancing professional knowledge' by academically respectable means (Golby and Parrott, 1999, p. 65). Yin (1994), argues that case study involves practice rather than philosophical enquiry. Golby and Parrott draw from this, three important points. These are that case study is an approach to research and not a method, that within this approach it is 'an open question what methods are to be used', and that it is not necessarily only qualitative methods that are acceptable. They argue rather that 'methods should be dictated by the need to understand, not selected on doctrinal grounds', (Golby and Parrott, 1999, p.66). They also argue that 'case study is appropriate where it is not yet clear what are the right questions to ask'. In these terms too, case study seems an appropriate approach for the kind of practitioner research with a practical enquiry thrust that we have in mind. This is because it involves a practitioner exploring in depth his or her own practice in such a way that it is very likely that the really important questions endemic to it will arise only at the end of the study (Golby and Parrott, 1999, p.66).

Golby and Parrott also argue that the case being studied must be conceived of as an example of *something*, and note the importance of seeing case study as the study of particularity rather than of uniqueness. In understanding a case it is necessary to see it within, and relate it in some way to, a wider context. It is only because it is possible to see it as an example of a general case that it is possible to say anything about it at all. If a case or incident within it were *unique*, such that nothing like it had ever been seen, it would be impossible to see to what it related, and thus impossible to make sense of it, beyond staring at it in wonder.

It should, of course be noted that case study research is very different from a patient case, the one being educational, the other medical, and each with its own focus and purpose, as the following table shows.

Table 11:3 Clinical case history and case study research.

Factors	Clinical case history	Case study research
Focus	Patient	Practitioner looks at own practice
Who does it?	Trainee surgeon	Practitioner (teacher/learner/doctor)
Purpose	To learn about medical condition X and the written evidence for its management	To understand better an aspect of one's own practice
Process	Review the medical literature about condition X Describe a series of medical conditions and interventions for Patient Y	Start with a critical incident (NOT a near miss) See below
Theory and practice	Use formal theory to critique specific practice	Theory and practice are mutually critical (each should critique the other)
Outcome	Improved and extended medical propositional knowledge only	Develops one's practice in the light of new understanding

A critical incident, as used within educational research can be the starting point for an educational enquiry. This can be a significant event with major consequences or a commonplace event that happened during routine practice, and that one suddenly became aware of, or came to see in a new light. Incidents are rendered critical by means of their analysis, interpretation and appreciation. They help us to see more in, and be more aware of, the detail of our practice

Equipped with these understandings, we now offer the following five brief suggestions for how to start on this process, following Fish and Coles, (1998), pp. 73-4.

1.   The homing-in process. This consists of identifying an issue or aspect of one's own practice and considering for whom it is important and why (there may be several answers to this).

2. Crystallizing the issue or problem. This consists of capturing a critical incident that is centrally associated with or illustrative of the issue, and analyzing and interpreting it, looking particularly at the values embedded in it, clarifying the context in which the incident arose and considering it carefully in the same way.

3. Identifying the nature of the issue or problem by examining the kinds of questions it engenders and thinking about it critically.

4. Investigating the matter further, both practically and theoretically by exploring your on-going practice and its practical and theoretical perspectives.

5. Making meaning out of the entire activity and planning for the future by engaging in analysis, interpretation and appreciation (see page 242).

It will readily be seen that practitioner research that uses a case study approach has much in common with that which uses an action research approach, but that the emphasis here is rather more centrally on changing practice and how to change it, rather than on the more modest illuminative intention of case study. Such approaches can also of course be used to complement each other. The important thrust is that the focus is one's own practice. Action research processes can be broadly characterized as follows.

❏ Review own current practice.
❏ Identify an aspect that needs improvement.
❏ Imagine a way forward.
❏ Try it out.
❏ Take stock of what happens.
❏ Modify action plan in the light of what is discovered and then continue with the action.
❏ Evaluate the modified action.
❏ Continue until satisfied with that aspect of own practice.

(adapted from McNiff, *et al*, 1996)

There is, of course, no 'right' way to go about practitioner research, but only that which is appropriate and best for the given situation. Professional judgement comes in here too!

Some helpful texts

We believe that the following references are particularly useful for surgeons who wish to pursue these matters.

On practitioner research generally

Fish, D. (1998) *Appreciating Practice in the Caring Professions: Re-focusing Professional Development and Practitioner Research.* Oxford: Butterworth Heinemann.
Pring, R. (2000) *Philosophy of Educational Research.* London: Continuum Books.

On case study research

Bassey, M. (1999) *Case Study Research in Educational Settings.* Buckingham: Open University Press.

Fish, D. and Coles, C. (1998) *Developing Professional Judgement in Health Care: learning through the critical appreciation of practice.* Oxford: Butterworth Heinemann.

Golby, M. and Parrott, A. (1999) *Educational Research and Educational Practice.* Exeter: Fair Way Press.

Stake, R. (1995) *The Art of Case Study Research.* London: Sage Publications

Yin, R. (1994) *Case Study Research: Design and Methods.* Newbury Park California: Sage Publications, (Second Edition).

On action research

Carr, W. and Kemmis, S. (1986) *Becoming Critical: Education, Knowledge and Action Research.* London: Falmer Press.

Elliott, J. (1991) *Action Research for Educational Change.* Buckingham: Open University Press.

McNiff, J., Lomax, P. and Whitehead, J. (1996) *You and your Action Research Project.* London: Routledge.

McNiff, J. with Whitehead, J. (2002) *Action research: Principles and Practice.* London: Routledge / Falmer, (Second Edition).

On the use of narrative in research

Fish, D. and Coles, C. (1998) *Developing Professional Judgement in Health Care: learning through the critical appreciation of practice.* Oxford: Butterworth Heinemann.

Greenhalgh, P. and Hurwitz, B. (1998) *Narrative Based Medicine: dialogue and discourse in clinical practice.* London: British Medical Journal Books.

Mason, J. (2002) *Researching Your Own Practice: The Discipline of Noticing.* London: Routledge/Falmer.

White, S. and Stancombe, J. (2003) *Clinical Judgement in the Health and Welfare Professions: extending the evidence base.* Maidenhead: Open University Press.

On discourse in medicine generally

Atkinson, P. (1995) *Medical Talk and Medical Work.* London: Sage Publications.

McLure, M. (2003) *Discourse in Educational and Social Research.* Buckingham: Open University Press.

Mishler, E.G. (1984) *The Discourse of Medicine: Dialectics of Medical Interviews.* Norwood, New Jersey: Ablex Publishing Corporation.

White, S. and Stancombe, J. (2003) *Clinical Judgement in the Health and Welfare Professions: extending the evidence base.* Maidenhead: Open University Press.

On Conversation Analysis

Hutchby, I. and Woolfitt, R. (1988/reprinted 2004) *Conversation Analysis.* Cambridge: Polity Press.

Ten Have, P. (1999) *Doing conversation analysis: a practical guide.* London: Sage Publications.

Final end note

We hope that readers will enjoy working further on teaching and learning in these ways, and can do no better than to quote the final paragraph of Fish and Twinn, (1997) in respect of this.

'There is always more to do and more to learn. Quality in patient and client care is not achieved by decree nor by striving to reach standards set by others, which are frequently raised before we can reach them. Rather it is achieved by the endless pursuit, by each practitioner, of greater understanding and better practice.'

(Fish and Twinn, 1997, p.181)

Index

A

U

References

Atkinson, P. (1995) *Medical Talk and Medical Work*. London: Sage Publications.

Bassey, M. (1999) *Case Study Research in Educational Settings*. Buckingham: Open University Press.

Benjamin, H. (1939) The Sabre-tooth Curriculum, in M. Golby, J. Greenwald, and R. West (eds.) (1975) *Curriculum Design*. London: Croom Helm in association with Open University Press.

Benner, P. (1984) *From Novice to Expert: Excellence and power in Clinical Nursing Practice*. London: Addison Wesley Publishing Company.

Bloom, B. S. (ed.) (1956) *Taxonomy of Educational Objectives: Handbook 1: The Cognitive Domain*. New York: David McKay and Co.

Bleakley, A. (2002) 'Pre-registration House Officers and ward-based learning: a new apprenticeship model', *Medical Education*, **36** (1): 1-9.

Bolton, G. (2001) *Reflective Practice: Writing and professional development*. London: Paul Chapman.

Boud, D., Keogh, R. and Walker, D. (eds.) (1985) *Reflection: Turning experience into learning*. London: Kogan Page.

Brigley, S., Golby, M., Johnson, C., *et al*, (2003) Report of an evaluation of the pilot project: Implementing The General Professional Practice in Surgery, paper presented to the RCS England, October 29th, 2003.

Brigley, S., Golby, M. and Robbé, I. (2004) 'The educational evaluation of The General Professional Practice of Surgery (GPPS)', *Annals of the Royal College of Surgeons of England*, **86** (9): 385-387.

Britton, N. (2004) 'Patients' expectations of Consultations', *British Medical Journal*, **328**, 21st Feb: 416-7.

Broadfoot, P. (1993) 'Educational Assessment: the myth of measurement'. Inaugral lecture given at the University of Bristol, on 25.10.1993. In P. Woods (ed.) (1996) *Contemporary issues in teaching and learning*. London: Routledge in association with the Open University, pp. 203-230.

Broadfoot, P. (2000) Assessment and Intuition, in T. Atkinson, and G. Claxton, (eds.) *The Intuitive Practitioner: on the value of not always knowing what one is doing.* Buckingham: Open University Press.

Brookfield, S. (2002) Clinical Reasoning and generic thinking skills, in J. Higgs, and M. Jones (eds.) *Clinical Reasoning in the Health Professions.* Oxford: Butterworth Heinemann, (Second Edition), 62-67.

Buckley, E. G. (1995) 'Apprentices or Spinning Tops - rotational programmes in postgraduate education?', *Medical Education*, **29**: 391-392.

Burke, J.W. (ed.) (1989) *Competency Based Education and Training.* London: The Falmer Press.

Carper, B. (1978) 'Fundamental Patterns of Knowing in Nursing', *Advances in Nursing Science*, **1**: 13-23.

Carr, D. (1993) 'Questions of Competence', *British Journal of Educational Studies*, **41**: 253-271.

Carr, W. (1995) *For Education: Towards Critical Educational Inquiry.* Buckingham: Open University Press.

Carr, W. and Kemmis, S. (1986) *Becoming Critical: Education, Knowledge and Action Research.* London: Falmer Press.

Chang, R.W., Bordage, G., and Connell, K.J. (1998) 'The importance of early problem representation during case presentations', *Academic Medicine*, **73** (10 suppl): 109-111.

Chikwe J, de Souza, A. and Pepper J. (2004) 'No time to train the surgeons'. *British Medical Journal,* **328**, 21st February: 418-19.

Cohn, E. (1989) 'Fieldwork Education: Shaping a foundation for Clinical Reasoning', *American Journal of Occupational Therapy*, **43** (4): 240-245.

Coles, C. (2000) Developing our intuitive knowing: an alternative approach to the assessment of doctors. In P. Bashook, S. Miller, J. Parboosingh, and S. Horowitz (Eds). *Credentialing Physician Specialists: A World Perspective.* Chicago: The Royal College of Physicians and Surgeons of Canada, and The American Board of Medical Specialties (June 2000).

Collins, J., Harkin, J, and Nind, M. (2002) *Manifesto for Learning.* London: Continuum Books.

Cotton, A. (2001) 'Private thoughts in public spheres: issues in reflection and reflective practices in nursing', *Journal of Advanced Nursing*, **36**: 512-519.

Cox, K. (1999) *Doctor and Patient: exploring clinical thinking.* Sydney: University of New South Wales Press.

Culshaw, H. (1995) 'Evidence-based practice for Sale?' *British Journal of Occupational Therapy*, **57**: 233.

Davies, C. (1998) Care and the Transformation of Professionalism, in T. Knijn and S. Sevenhuijsen (eds.) *Care, Citizenship and Social Cohesion.* Utrecht: Netherlands School of Social and Economic Policy Research. (Also, abridged in: C. Davies, L. Findlay and A. Bullman (eds.) (2000) *Changing Practice in Health and Social Care.* London: Open University in association with Sage Publications: 343-354.

de Cossart, L., Wiltshire, C., and Brown, J. (2001) 'An audit of the operative skills of SHOs on a Basic Surgical Training Programme', *Annals of the Royal College of Surgeons (Supplement)*, **83** (11): 326-327.

de Cossart L. and Fish, D. (2002) 'Membership of a Profession: Part Two: The nature of professional knowledge in medical clinical practice', *Mersey Deanery Newsletter* **14**, (2), Liverpool: Mersey Deanery for PGMDE.

Department of Health and Social Security, (2002) *Unfinished Business.* London: Her Majesty's Stationery Office (www.doh.gov.uk).

Department of Health and Social Security, (2003) *Modernising Medical Careers.* London: Her Majesty's Stationery Office (www.doh.gov.uk).

Department of Health and Social Security, (2004) MMC The next steps - The future shape of Foundation, *Specialist and General Practice Training Programmes.* London: Her Majesty's Stationery Office (*www.doh.gov.uk*).

Dewey, J. (1897) 'My pedagogic creed', *The School Journal.* **LIV** (3): Jan 16 1897: 77-80 (*http://www.infed.org/archives/e-texts/e-dew-pc.htm*).

Dewey, J. (1910, revised edition 1933), *How We Think.* New York: Dover Publications Inc.

Dewey, J. (1916) *Democracy and Education.* New York: Free Press.

Dowie, J. and Elstein, A. (eds.) (1988) *Professional Judgement: A Reader in Clinical Decision-making.* Cambridge: Cambridge University Press.

Downie, R.S. and Macnaughton, J. (2000) *Clinical Judgement: Evidence in practice.* Oxford: Oxford University Press.

Driscoll, J. (2000) *Practising Clinical Supervision: a reflective approach.* Edinburgh: Ballière Tindall and the Royal College of Nursing.

Elliott, J. (1991) *Action research for educational change.* Buckingham: Open University Press.

Epstein, R.M. (1999) 'Mindful Practice', *Journal of the American Medical Association*, **282** (9): 282-283.

Eraut, M. (1994) *Developing Professional Knowledge and Competence*. London: The Falmer Press.

Eraut, M. (1995) 'Schön Shock: a case for re-framing reflection in action?' *Teachers and Training: Theory and Practice*, **1** (1): 9-23.

Eraut (1998) 'Concepts of Competence', *Competence to Practice Volume of Journal of Inter-professional Care*, **12** (2): 127-141.

Eraut, M. (2001) 'Editorial' in *Learning in Health and Social Care*, **2** (1): 1-4.

Eraut, M. and du Boulay, B. (2000) Developing the Attributes of Medical Professional Judgement and Competence. Brighton: University of Sussex. (http://www.cogs.susx.ac.uk/users/bend/doh/reporthmtl.hmtl).

Fish, D. (1995) *Quality Mentoring for Student Teachers: A Principled Approach to Practice*. London: David Fulton.

Fish, D. (1998) *Appreciating Practice in the Caring Professions: Re-focusing Professional Development and Practitioner Research*. Oxford: Butterworth Heinemann.

Fish, D. (2003) Education in a community of professional practice: a new approach to curriculum design, in *Report of Research for Cancer Research-UK on a base line of education for Cancer Care*. London: Cancer Research-UK.

Fish, D. (2004) 'The Educational Thinking behind the Royal College of Surgeons of England's First Curriculum Framework', *Annals of the Royal College of Surgeons of England*, **86** (7): 312-315.

Fish, D. (2005) The Anatomy of Evaluation, in M. Rose, and D. Best (eds.) *Understanding Supervision in Health Science Education and Practice*. Edinburgh: Elsevier (forthcoming August 2005).

Fish, D., and Coles. C. (eds.) (1998) *Developing Professional Judgement in Health Care: Learning through the critical appreciation of practice*. Oxford: Butterworth-Heinemann.

Fish, D. and Coles, C. (2005) *Medical Education: Developing a Curriculum for Practice*. Maidenhead: Open University Press in association with McGraw Hill, (forthcoming).

Fish, D. and Twinn, S. (1997) *Quality Clinical Supervision in the Health Care Professions: Principled Approaches to Practice*. Oxford: Butterworth Heinemann.

Fish, D., Twinn, S. and Purr, B. (1989) H*ow to enable Learning Through Professional Practice*. London: West London Press.

Freidson, E. (1994) *Professionalism Reborn: Theory, Prophecy and Policy*. Oxford: Polity Press.

Freidson, E. (2001) *Professionalism: the Third Way.* Oxford: Polity Press.

Freshwater, D. (ed.) (2002) *Therapeutic Nursing: improving patient care through self-awareness and reflection.* London: Sage Publications.

Gardner, H. (1993) *Frames of Mind.* New York: Basic Books.

Gawande, A. (2001) *Complications: A Surgeon's notes on an Imperfect Science.* London: Profile Books.

Gibbs, G. (1988) *Learning by Doing. A Guide to Teaching and Learning Methods.* Further Education Unit, Oxford Polytechnic, Oxford.

Glass, R.D. (1996) *Diagnosis: a brief introduction.* Melbourne: Oxford University Press.

General Medical Council (1999) *The doctor as Teacher.* London: GMC.

General Medical Council (2001) *Good Medical Practice.* London: GMC.

Golby, M. (1993) 'Educational Research' in *Educational Research: Trick or Treat?* Exeter Society for Curriculum Studies, **15** (3): 5-8.

Golby, M. and Parrott, A. (1999) *Educational Research and Educational Practice.* Exeter: Fair Way Press.

Grant, J. and Marsden, P. (1988) 'Primary Knowledge, medical education and consultant expertise', *Medical Education,* **22** (3): 173-179.

Greenhalgh, P. and Hurwitz, B. (1998) *Narrative Based Medicine: dialogue and discourse in clinical practice.* London: BMJ Books.

Greenwood, J. (1993) 'Reflective Practice: a critique of the work of Argyris and Schön', *Journal of Advanced Nursing,* **18**: 1183-1187.

Grundy, S. (1987) *The Curriculum: Product or Praxis.* London: The Falmer Press.

Habermas, J. (1971) *Towards a Rational Society.* Trans. J.J. Shappiro, London: Heinemann.

Habermas, J. (1972) *Knowledge and Human Interest.* Trans. J.J. Shappiro, London: Heinemann.

Habermas, J. (1974) *Theory and Practice.* Trans, J. Viertel, London: Heinemann.

Higgs, J . (1990) 'Fostering the Acquisition of Clinical reasoning skills', *New Zealand Journal of Occupational Therapy,* December 1990: 13-18.

Higgs, J. (2003) Do you reason like a (health) professional? In G. Brown, S. Esdaile, and S. Ryan (eds.) *Becoming an Advanced Practitioner.* Edinburgh: Butterworth Heinemann (145-160).

Higgs, J., Andressen, A. and Fish, D. (2004) Practice knowledge - its nature sources and contexts, in J. Higgs, B. Richardson and M. Abrandt Dahlgren (eds.) *Developing Practice Knowledge for Health Professionals*. Edinburgh: Butterworth Heinemann.

Higgs, J., Fish, D. and Rothwell, R. (2004) Practice knowledge - critical appreciation. In J. Higgs, B. Richardson, and M. Abrandt Dahlgren (eds.) *Developing Practice Knowledge for Health Professionals*. Edinburgh: Butterworth Heinemann.

Higgs, J. and Jones, M. (eds.) (2002) *Clinical Reasoning in the Health Professions*. Oxford: Butterworth Heinemann, (Second Edition).

Higgs, J., Jones, M., Edwards, I. and Beeston, S (2004) Clinical reasoning and knowledge practice, Chapter 11, in J. Higgs, B. Richardson, M. and Abrandt Dahlgren (eds) *Developing Practice Knowledge for Health Professionals*. Edinburgh: Butterworth Heinemann.

Higgs, J. and Titchen, A. (2001) Knowledge and Reasoning, in J. Higgs, and M. Jones (eds.) (2002) *Clinical Reasoning in the Health Professions*. Oxford: Butterworth Heinemann, (Second Edition).

Hoyle, E. (1974) 'Professionality, professionalism and the control of teaching', *London Educational Review*, **3** (2): 3-18.

Hutchby, I. and Woolfitt, R. (1988/reprinted 2004) *Conversation Analysis*. Cambridge: Polity Press.

Johns, C. (2002) *Guided Reflection: advancing practice*. Oxford: Blackwell Publishing.

Kassirer, J.P. and Kopelman, R. I. (1991) *Learning Clinical Reasoning*. Baltimore, MD: Williams and Wilkins.

Katory M., Singh, S. and Beard J.D. (2001) 'Twenty Trent trainees: a comparison of operative competence after BST'. *Annals of the Royal College of Surgeons of England (Suppl)*, **83**: 328-330.

Kirk, R.M. and Cox, K. (2004) Decision making, in R.M. Kirk, and W.J. Ribbans, (eds.) *Clinical Surgery in General*. London: Churchill Livingstone, (Fourth Edition).

Kolb, D. (1984) *Experiential Learning as the science of learning and development*. Englewood Cliffs, New Jersey: Prentice Hall.

Krathwohl, D.R., Bloom, B.S. and Masia, B.B. (1964) *Taxonomy of Educational Objectives: Handbook II: The Affective Domain*. New York: McKay.

Lamond, D., Crow, R. and Chase, J. (1996) 'Judgements and processes in care decisions in acute medical and surgical wards', *Journal of Evaluation in Clinical Practice*. **2** (3): 211-216.

Macdonald, M. (1997) Craft Knowledge in Medicine: An Interpretation of Teaching and Learning in Apprenticeship. Unpublished PhD thesis, Open University.

Mason, J. (2002) *Researching Your Own Practice: The Discipline of Noticing.* London: Routledge/Falmer.

Mattingly, C. and Fleming, M. (1994) *Clinical Reasoning: Forms of Inquiry in Therapeutic Practice.* Philadelphia: F. A. Davis Co.

McLure, M. (2003) *Discourse in Educational and Social Research.* Buckingham: Open University Press.

McNiff, J., Lomax, P. and Whitehead, J. (1996) *You and Your Action Research Project.* London: Routledge.

McNiff, J. with Whitehead, J. (2002) *Action Research: Principles and practice.* London: Routledge/Falmer, (Second edition).

Mishler, E.G. (1984) *The Discourse of Medicine: Dialectics of Medical Interviews.* Norwood, New Jersey: Ablex Publishing Corporation.

Moon, J. (1999) *Reflection in Learning and Professional Development: Theory and Practice.* London: Kogan Page.

Newble, D. and Cannon, R. (1994) *A Handbook for Medical Teachers.* Edinburgh: Elsevier.

Oakeshott, M. (1967) *On Human Conduct.* Oxford: Clarendon Books.

O'Neill, O. (2002) *A Question of Trust.* Cambridge: Cambridge University Press. (The 2002 Reith Lectures).

Patel, V.A. and Groen, G.J. (1986) 'Knowledge based solution strategies in medical reasoning', *Cognitive Science*, **10**: 91-116.

Pereira Grey, D. (2002) 'Deprofessionalising doctors?' *British Medical Journal*, **324**: 627-8.

Phenix, P. H. (1964) *Realms of Meaning.* New York: McGraw-Hill.

Playdon, Z. J. (2004) 'The Management Evaluation of General Professional Practice [in] Surgery (GPPS)', *Annals of the Royal College of Surgeons of England*, **86** (9): 387-390.

Pring, R. (2000) *Philosophy of Educational Research.* London: Continuum Books.

Proctor, B. (1986) Supervision: a cooperative exercise in accountability, in M. Marken, and M. Paynes, (eds.) *Enabling and Ensuring - supervision in practice.* Leicester: National Youth Bureau, Council for Education and Training in Youth and Community Work: 21-34.

Richardson, B., Higgs J. and Abrandt Dahlgren, M. (2004) Recognising practice epistemology in the health professions, in J. Higgs, B. Richardson, and M. Abrandt Dahlgren, (eds.) *Developing Practice Knowledge for Health Professionals*. Edinburgh: Butterworth Heinemann.

Ridderikhoff, J. (1991) 'Medical problem-solving: an exploration of strategies', *Medical Education*, **25**: 106-107.

Rimoldi, H. J. (1988) 'Diagnosing the diagnostic process', *Medical Education*, **22**: 270-278.

Rolfe, G. (ed) (2000) *Nursing praxis and the reflexive practitioner: collected papers 1993-1999*. London: Nursing Praxis International.

Rose, M. and Best, D. (eds.) (2005) *Understanding Supervision in Health Science Education and Practice*. Edinburgh: Elsevier, (due August 2005).

Royal College of Surgeons of England, (1996) *The Manual of Basic Surgical Training (The Blue Book)*. London: Royal College of Surgeons of England.

Royal College of Surgeons of England, (2001) A College Curriculum for Basic Surgical Training: How People Learn and the Values that Motivate them: a first announcement. October 2001, London: Royal College of Surgeons of England.

Royal College of Surgeons of England (2002), *Good Surgical Practice*. London: Royal College of Surgeons of England.

Royal College of Surgeons of England, (2003) The General Professional Practice of Surgery Draft Curriculum for SHO Education. London: Royal College of Surgeons of England (September 2003).

Ryan, S. (1995) Teaching Reasoning to Occupational Therapists during Fieldwork Education, in J. Higgs, and M. Jones (eds.) *Clinical Reasoning in the Health Professions*. (First Edition). Oxford: Butterworth Heinemann.

Ryan, S., Esdale, S. and Brown, G. (2003) Appreciating the Big Picture: you are part of it! In G. Brown, S. Esdaile, and S. Ryan (eds.) *Becoming an Advanced Practitioner.* Edinburgh: Butterworth Heinemann.

Ryle, G. (1949) *The Concept of Mind*. Harmonsdsworth: Penguin.

Sackett, D.L., Richardson, S., Rosenburg, W. and Haynes, R.B. (1997) *Evidence-based Medicine: how to practise and teach it*. Edinburgh: Churchill Livingstone.

Saks, M. (1998) Professionalism and Health Care, in S. Taylor and D. Field, (eds.) *Sociological Perspectives on Health, Illness and Health Care*. Oxford: Blackwell Science. (Also, abridged in: C. Davies, L. Findlay and A. Bullman (eds.) (2000) *Changing Practice in Health and Social Care*. London: Open University in association with Sage Publications).

Schmidt, H.G. and Boshuizen, H.P.A. (1993) 'On acquiring expertise in medicine'. *Educational Psychology Review*, **5** (3): 205-221.

Schmidt, H.G., Boshuizen, H.P.A. and Norman, G.R. (1992) Reflection on the nature of expertise in Medicine, in E. Keravnou (ed.) *Deep Models of Medical Knowledge Engineering*, Amsterdam: Elsevier: 231-248.

Schön, D. (1983) *The Reflective Practitioner*. New York: Basic Books.

Schön, D. (1987) *Educating the Reflective Practitioner*. New York: Jossey Bass.

Schön, D (ed.) (1991) *The Reflective Turn: case studies in and on educational practice*. New York: The Teachers College Press.

Sefton, A., Gordon, J. and Field, M. (2002) Teaching Clinical Reasoning to medical students, in J. Higgs, and M. Jones, (eds.) *Clinical Reasoning in the Health Professions*. Oxford: Butterworth Heinemann, (Second Edition).

Shah, Z. (2003) 'Endpiece', *British Medical Journal*, **327**, 29th Nov: 1263.

Southern, G. and Braithwaite, J. (1998) 'The End of Professionalism?' in *Social Science and Medicine,* **46** (1): 23-28. (Also, abridged in: C. Davies, L. Findlay and A. Bullman (eds.) (2000) *Changing Practice in Health and Social Care*. London: Open University in association with Sage Publications: 300-307.)

Stake, R. (1995) *The Art of Case Study Research*. London: Sage Publications.

Stenhouse, L. (1975) *An Introduction to Curriculum Research and Development*. London: Heinemann.

Stiwne, D. and Abrandt Dahlgren, M. (2004) Challenging evidence in evidence-based practice, in J. Higgs, B. Richardson, and M. Abrandt Dahlgren (eds.) *Developing Practice Knowledge for Health Professionals*. Edinburgh: Butterworth Heinemann.

Stones, E. (1979) *Psychopedagogy: psychological theory and the practice of teaching*. London: Methuen and Co Ltd.

Talbot, M. (2004) 'Monkey see, monkey do: a critique of the competency model in graduate medical education', *Medical Education*, **38**: 587-592.

Ten Have, P. (1999) *Doing conversation analysis: a practical guide*. London: Sage Publications.

Thompson, C. and Dowding, D. (eds) (2002) *Clinical Decision Making and Judgement in Nursing*. London: Churchill Livingstone.

Tripp, D. (1993) *Critical Incidents in Teaching: Developing Professional Judgement*. London: Routledge.

Tyler, R. (1949) *Basic Principles of Curriculum and Instruction*. Chicago: Chicago University Press.

Vallis, J., Hesketh, A. and MacPherson, S. (2004) 'Pre-registration house officer training: a role for nurses in the new Foundation Programme?' *Medical Education*, **38**, (7): 708-716.

Van Manen, M. (1977) 'Linking ways of knowing with ways of being', *Curriculum Inquiry*, **6**: 205-88.

Van Manen, M. (1991) *The Tact of Teaching*. New York: The State of New York Press.

Wells, G. (1986/2002) Conversation and the Re-invention of Knowledge, in A. Pollard. (ed.) *Readings for Reflective Teaching*. London: Continuum Books.

Wenger, E. (1999) *Communities of Practice: Leaning, Meaning and Identity*. Cambridge: Cambridge University Press.

West, L. (2001) *Doctors on the Edge: General Practitioners, Health and Learning in the Inner City*. London: Free Association Books.

White, S. and Stancombe, J. (2003) *Clinical Judgement in the Health and Welfare Professions: extending the evidence base*. Maidenhead: Open University Press.

Winter, R., Buck, A. and Sobiechowska, P. (1999) *Professional Experience and the investigative imagination: the ART of reflective writing*. London: Routledge.

Wolf, A. (1995) *Competence-based Assessment*. London: Open University Press.

Wragg, E. (1994) 'Look on my works ye mighty, and despair', *Times Educational Supplement*, 25th November.

Yin, R. (1994) *Case Study Research: Design and Methods*. Newbury Park, California: Sage Publications, (Second Edition).